D1571808

Functional Fitness

Look Younger, Stay Active Longer

Paul D'Arezzo, M.D.

Illustrations by Nathanael Letteer

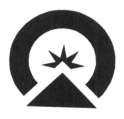

Marcellina Mountain Press
Colorado Springs, Colorado

For my mother,
who always encouraged my writing

About the Author

Paul D'Arezzo, MD, is a board-certified emergency physician having practiced in Florida, Hawaii, and Colorado. Over the years after seeing countless patients with muscle and joint complaints, he became acutely aware that there are things we can do to prevent or at least forestall much of the muscle and joint pain and disability commonly associated with aging. Combining his extensive medical background with yoga and other disciplines, he presents a clear case for the need to take an active role in staying young and active. Currently retired from active practice, he resides in Colorado Springs, Colorado where he devotes much of his time and energy to spreading this message.

Acknowledgments

- My wife, Rebecca, for all her encouragement and support.

- Pete Egoscue and The Egoscue Method for opening my eyes to the importance of body alignment.

- Nate Letteer for his wonderful illustrations.

- To my yoga teachers—Namaste.

Disclaimer: This book is not a substitute for professional healthcare and makes no claims and takes no responsibility for the results any given individual may obtain by following the prescribed advice or exercise programs. If you are an older individual or have any underlying medical conditions, it is always prudent to seek the advice of your doctor or healthcare provider before initiating any exercise program. As always, listen to your own body and use your own best judgment.

© Paul D'Arezzo 2005

All rights reserved. No part of this book may be reproduced or transmitted in any form or by any means, electronic or mechanical, including photocopying, recording, or by any information or storage retrieval system, without written permission from the author, except for the use of brief quotations in review articles.

Published by Marcellina Mountain Press
               P.O. Box 6781
               Colorado Springs, CO 80934

Website: www.posturealignment.com

Illustrations by Nathanael Letteer

Layout and Design by Paige Ink

ISBN 0-9729079-1-2

Library of Congress Control Number: 2005926865

Printed by Hignell Book Printing in Canada

Contents

Introduction

On the day I turned forty, I remember an older doctor coming up to me and saying "After forty, everything is downhill." His comment bothered me. I had always been physically active; I hiked and biked and played tennis. But already I was beginning to feel creaks in my knees, and it was getting harder to do simple things like bend down and pick up a piece of paper under a table or to get down on the floor and play with my kids.

I didn't want to hurt in my joints like so many of the patients I saw. I didn't want to live on a diet of Motrin™. I didn't want to look and move like my parents or grandparents long before I thought I should. At the very least I wanted to forestall and prevent those things as long as possible.

This made me curious—were all these changes I was experiencing simply the effects of aging? Or were there things we could do to prevent or forestall some of these changes in our muscle and joint health. More importantly were there things we were doing—or not doing—that were contributing to loss of muscle and joint function. This is how I became interested in functional fitness.

Most of us have long ago given up our dreams of becoming world-class figure skaters or playing in the Super Bowl. Our physical lives are more prosaic. We live our lives sitting down and standing up and reaching under tables for things that have fallen. We live our lives climbing stairs and reaching up to put our baggage in overhead compartments. We live our lives carrying groceries and climbing in and out of cars. We live our lives wanting to play with our kids without hurting or wanting to perhaps play a sport we like once or twice a week.

In a word, what we are after is function. We want to be able to do everything we want and need to do for as long as possible without muscle and joint pain or disability interfering. We want to stay active as long as possible. And we want to remain young-looking as long as we can. Much of looking older (no matter what age you pick for that) is based on our posture and how we move or don't move.

Even though I'm a doctor, I'm not going to tell you about the most recent research in arthritis or discuss the different types of joint replacement surgery. I'm not going to tell you to take a certain supplement. I'm not going to discuss the different classes of arthritis pain medications and their side effects or tell you how to shop around for the best orthopedist. I'll leave those things to others.

What I am going to do is give you something far simpler and cheaper, and something you intuitively already know. We, you and I, personally have a decided stake in staying functional. There are things we can do, that no doctor or health provider can do, to prevent and forestall some of the muscle and joint changes we commonly associate with aging.

This book draws us back to our roots. Something is often forgotten, overlooked, or glossed over in our rush for quick fixes, miracle drugs, and surgery. My goal is to increase your awareness on the importance of four things: staying strong, staying flexible, correcting and maintaining your posture, and staying active. My foremost goal is to present you with principles that will serve you well into your advancing years.

This book also contains exercises. Most of us have neither the time nor inclination to spend long hours in a gym jumping up and down off small steps to lively music or lifting massive weights above our heads. The exercises in this book are specifically designed to target the areas most susceptible to changing with aging. They work. Try any or all of the exercises. They *will* make a difference in your life. You will feel better. You will feel stronger, healthier, and more vibrant; and you will look younger. Pains that have been bothering you for a long time may very well go away. Sometimes only a small improvement in strength, flexibility, or body alignment is enough to take pressure off an area that is being rubbed raw, or provide relief for muscles that have been going into spasm. Doing something *now* can be enough to prevent the onset or progression of certain types of arthritis or the need for joint replacement surgery in the future.

The exercises in this book will bring a surge of energy into your life. They will make you feel, physically, that you can and want to do more. They may prevent you from giving up a sport or activity you may have thought it was time to give up. Or they may encourage you to take up a new one.

This book makes no claims on making you ageless. Truly, there are no survivors on this earth. But if we can enjoy and carry out our life's responsibilities without pain or disability, if we can remain functional and active longer into our later years, then that is surely something worthwhile.

CHAPTER 1

You Don't Know What You've Got Until It's Gone

Don't it always seem to go
That you don't know what you've got til it's gone.

—Joni Mitchell, "Big Yellow Taxi"

Our bodies are our intimate partners. Unfortunately, our friends and spouses may desert us, but our bodies invariably remain with us for better or worse, for richer or for poorer, and in sickness and in health.

Our quality of life is intimately connected with the functioning of our bodies. I don't need to tell you this if you've ever been gravely sick or suffer from some disability. Much of what we take for granted for years suddenly becomes a hardship. Simply getting around can require extreme effort. Even minor muscle and joint pain and disability can sap our strength and concentration.

We may very well be spiritual beings having a human experience, but until the day we die, we are and will remain animals. And as animals we are subject to the limitations, restrictions, and rules of these bodies.

This book is specifically about muscle and joint health. Our muscles and joints are the platform on which we play and live out our lives. They are what allow us to work, play, and carry out the host of other activities, both necessary and enjoyable, that make up our lives.

The premise of this book is that there are things we can do to prevent or at least to forestall much of the diminution in our muscle and joint functioning with age. Much of what we blame on simply aging not need occur, or at least not to the degree that it often does. A great deal of our joint pain, arthritis, muscle spasms, and low back problems can be prevented.

> Much of the muscle and joint pain and disability
> commonly associated with aging is preventable.

We Don't Break Down All At Once—It's A Gradual Process

Life gives us a grace period with regard to our bodies. For much of our lives, particularly when we are younger, our bodies work in the background like faithful servants doing our biding without question or complaint. They put up with our weekend warrior attempts, our long periods of inactivity, and our days, weeks, and years of repetitive activity.

But then after a certain point, often after a certain age, our muscles and joints begin to make themselves known or rather felt. "The old back isn't what it used to be." "My knees go out." "It hurts to do that." "I don't want to do that anymore. It's no fun." "Park the car closer; I don't want to walk that far!"

We often think these things occur out of the blue, but more often they are the result of a slow progressive loss of function. It is only when things reach a critical point that we become aware of what may have been going on beneath the surface for a long time.

Muscle and joint loss of function sneak up on us. They are insidious. We lose a bit here and a bit there. We become weaker and less flexible by degrees. We stop doing this and that. We stop playing a sport or doing an activity we used to love. Physical activities we used to do just don't seem fun anymore. We hire someone to do what we used to do ourselves.

And for long stretches of time, we may not do much of anything. Then suddenly we find that we are no longer able to do what we used to do.

> Loss of physical functioning sneaks up on us.

Or we begin to hurt—a twinge of pain here, a deep aching in our hip once in awhile, trouble supporting our weight fully on our left leg. (Will our knee give out? Is it arthritis? Maybe it will go away.)

With time the twinge of pain becomes a constant ache. We begin to *always* favor using our right side to support us and develop an imbalance in our walk, or our hips or knees begin to bother us almost all the time.

> Small pains become big pains. Occasional pain becomes constant pain.

We visit doctors and get X-rays. We take pain medications. Maybe we have chiropractic adjustments. But with time, the pain comes back in the same place or another place. And because of the pain we become less active or gain weight, both of which contribute to a further decrease in our muscle and joint functioning. We fall prey to an ever-increasing spiral of decreased activity. We become disabled to greater or lesser degrees. Something we just have to live with. Maybe.

> Pain leads to decreased activity and a further decrease in function.

For many people, this insidious loss of function, the muscle and joint pain and the subsequent disability is happening at younger and younger ages—twenties, thirties, forties.

But we often don't become fully conscious of the degradation of our physical functioning until something dramatic happens and draws our attention to it. Often it takes an injury, having to be off work, chronic pain, or giving up an activity that we really love for us to wake up and take notice.

The rust that has been eating its way through the muffler of our car has been going on a long time before the muffler finally breaks loose and starts banging underneath the car. In the same way, the deterioration in our muscle and joint health has often been going on a long time before it reaches a critical point and we notice it. Something often has to break or begin hurting fulltime to garner our full attention.

> Pains and injuries that seemingly occur out of the blue are often the end result of a long progression of deterioration in our muscle and joint health that has been going on beneath the surface for a long time.

It would be a blessing if perhaps an idiot light came on on our foreheads well before injury or disability occurred, and that we be demanded to pull over and take care of things before being allowed to move on.

But our bodies aren't like that. We are allowed to continue to function with and in spite of growing under-the-surface muscle and joint deterioration.

Some of us wake up with these wake-up calls. We do something about it. We begin exercising and taking an active role in maintaining our muscle and joint health.

Some of us don't know exactly what to do. We see and feel the changes in our muscles and joints but don't know what to do or if there is any way to stop it. And some of us simply accept it, begrudgingly at first, as simple aging—a fact of life. After all, my father began having back pain about this age. Or my aunt has had knee replacement surgery, and she is younger than I am. We may wonder, however, in the back of our minds, "If this is the way things are now, what are they going to be like years from now?"

> There are things we can do to prevent or forestall much of the deterioration in our muscle and joint health.

The Downward Spiral

In medicine, a physician is always vigilant to prevent any small insult to the body from expanding. As a doctor, once you get behind the eight ball with a patient, it can become increasingly hard to turn things around. A patient in the ICU with heart problems is prone to electrolyte abnormalities, which may lead to an irregular heart beat. An irregular heart beat may lead to a fall in blood pressure. A fall in blood pressure may lead to the patient suffering respiratory problems and developing pneumonia. Antibiotics for the pneumonia may precipitate kidney problems. And on it goes.

> In medicine, we want to limit or curtail the first insults to an organ system before they have a chance to expand.

I call this cascading deterioration *the downward spiral*. It is the same with our muscles and joints, our musculoskeletal system. If we aren't careful, small seemingly insignificant chinks in our musculoskeletal armor spiral downward over time precipitating further deterioration in our musculoskeletal and overall health.

Here's an example. If through a sedentary lifestyle, we become weak in a key muscle group, increased pressure on one of our joints may result. Our knee or hip begins to hurt. We are less likely to be active. If we aren't active, other muscles become weak. Other muscles become stiff. Our posture begins to sag and collapse. A sagging posture often concentrates the weight of our body in one area, a hip or one side of our back. Now our back begins to hurt. We become even less active. We gain weight. We fall or twist something. Inactivity sets the stage for arthritis and a host of other diseases ... you get the idea. And down we go.

There are endless variations on the downward spiral. Any musculoskeletal compromise, while seemingly isolated, contributes to further compromise. The key initial common denominators, however, are often loss of muscular strength, loss of flexibility, and alterations in our body's posture or alignment. Here's another example of the downward spiral—

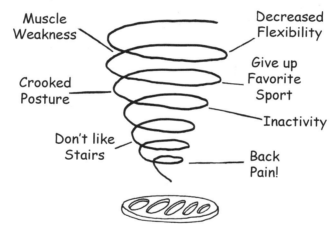

> We want to avoid and prevent the initial chinks in our musculoskeletal armor that allow the downward spiral to get started.

If you hurt now or suspect you are already somewhere on the continuum of the downward spiral, there are things you can do to limit your progression down the spiral or to step off of it. And if you feel fine, there are things you can do now to prevent and forestall your journey down the downward spiral. As the title of this chapter implies, we often take for granted our physical health until it begins to deteriorate. We don't notice things until they are gone. And then we look back and say,

"You know, compared to now, I was able to do quite a few things back then."

"If the shoe fits, the foot is forgotten," says the ancient sage. And it is only when the shoe doesn't fit—when our muscles and joints begin to hurt or give way—that we take notice. We take for granted all the things we *can* do now. We take for granted the places we *don't* hurt now. We want to keep it that way.

> It's human nature. We often don't notice or appreciate all the things that are right until they go wrong.

There May Not Be Much Left Of You When It Comes Time To Retire

It's a sobering thought. You may work all those years and *do everything right*, but then in the end your body fails you. You may not be able to play golf like you thought you would. Or you may not be able to take that trip with your spouse you always dreamed of; the physical demands of travel may be too much for you. Play golf, swim, hike, exercise, work around the house—maybe? Or even if you don't plan to be particularly active in retirement, will your retirement years be upset by chronic back pain or by hip pain, or a nagging disability that demands much of your attention.

A body that hurts becomes an intrusion in our lives. If it hurts every time you go up or down stairs, or have to bend down to pick something up, it siphons away your life energy. Even if retirement is still decades away, it's useful to ask the question: Are we doing what we can to assure a functional future?

Just as we prepare for our financial future, are we doing what we can to plan and prepare for our muscle and joint future?

How Modern Society Contributes To Loss Of Function

Modern society doesn't help. Most of us simply aren't required to physically do that much any more. We are very busy—busier than ever— but unfortunately we move in a few simple repetitive ways. We sit a lot. We sit in our cars, at our jobs, and back home on the couch. We aren't required to bend down, lift, or stretch as much as our ancestors. This relative lack of activity contributes to the downward spiral.

Technological advances, while marvelous, conspire to make us less active. We no longer *need* to physically do much anymore. Each new thing that does something for us, that requires us *not* to get up or to move, stretch, or reach, contributes to us falling prey to the downward spiral. And if we aren't careful, we become *no longer be able to do* things.

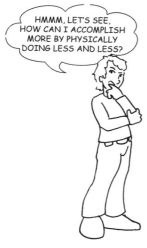

HMMM, LET'S SEE, HOW CAN I ACCOMPLISH MORE BY PHYSICALLY DOING LESS AND LESS?

Indeed, throughout history success or efficiency has been equated with accomplishing more and more while physically being required to do less and less.

More and more, many of us control our empires ensconced at our computer terminals or driving around with our cell phones pressed to our ears.

This diminution in physical activity is not without its cost however. Our heritage intervenes. Much as we try we can't hide our coarse upbringing, nor should we want to. We come from a long legacy of diggers, jumpers, walkers, hunters, and gatherers. Just as plants need light to grow, just as machinery needs lubrication to keep operating properly, we need a wide variety of movement to remain functional and to prevent many of our muscle and joint maladies. Movement is the juice that keeps our bodies functional.

> Unless we make a conscious effort to fight it, modern society contributes to a loss of function and makes us prone to the downward spiral.

> We need to move and to be active.

We might hope that it would be different, that we would outgrow this need to move and to keep our bodies functional, that the need to move might be relegated to children in school playgrounds or to professional athletes. But it's not, and it won't be.

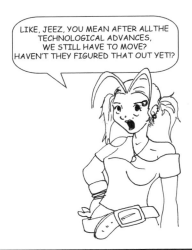

Our bodies follow a simple rule that can't be unseated: Use it or lose it. That which is not used deteriorates. This includes our muscles and joints.

What We're After—Functional Fitness

What we are after is a functional body that doesn't hurt, one that allows us to easily participate in a variety of activities, one that allows us to do all the things we enjoy and want to do for as long as possible.

What we are after is function.

This book's goal is to give you tools to preserve and maintain much of the function we need for daily living: getting in and out of cars, twisting, turning, picking things up off the floor, playing with our children or grandchildren, going up and down stairs, walking, carrying things, lifting things, doing stuff around the house, and continuing to participate in the sports and activities we love.

Our goal is to restore and maintain our muscle and joint health in order to allow us to keep doing as much as possible for as long as possible.

The Answer

The answer to the preservation of our physical function is not complicated. However, it may not be the quick-fix solution in three easy payments of $19.95 that we'd like to hear. It may take some effort and commitment. We may prefer a simpler, less-demanding solution. But let me clear this up right now—

> There is going to be no magic pill, no nutritional supplement, no chiropractic adjustment, no splint, no surgery, and no change in the level of your computer screen that is going to solve all your muscle and joint problems long term.

All these things may have their place, but it is backward thinking where they are often expected to cure us rather than be relegated to accessory positions. More often they are palliative at best.

Even orthopedic surgery, while miraculous, should be seen as a solution of last resort. It is not without complications. Can orthopedic surgery such as joint replacement surgery be lifesaving in terms of pain and mobility? Definitely, yes. But it is often backward thinking where we allow things to progress to the point where we need such drastic methods to fix us. Or when we don't even consider that we might have something to do with what's been going on.

Are there wonder-drugs that can help people with muscle and joint problems function with less pain and disability? Of course there are. But when we expect a drug to cure all our woes or become dependent on them without even considering reversible causes of our problems, that's where we need to think again.

We often have a bias toward complex, high-tech solutions to our problems, while simpler, commonsense solutions are given short shrift.

> The simplest solutions are often the best.

Too often we turn toward complex solutions too quickly and too early rather than addressing the simpler, obvious solutions: weakness, stiffness, loss of alignment, inactivity.

> We are often a little too quick to go to the medicine cabinet, to blame our problems on aging or arthritis, to demand surgery, or to expect someone or something else to fix us.

Accidents Happen

Accidents are just that—accidents. They happen. After years of working as an Emergency Room doctor, I know that bad things happen to everyone. No one is immune. No amount of healthy living or exercise can prevent injury from occurring sometimes.

But for many of our muscle and joint injuries in particular, we have a decided stake in them occurring. Just as we individually can take steps to prevent heart disease and a host of other diseases, similarly we can take steps that limit our propensity to muscle and joint injury and subsequent disability.

I have the utmost compassion for anyone who is injured or is in pain, but at the same time, it is often naïve to think we have nothing to do with preventing many of our injuries or disabilities. Weakness of muscles, stiffness of muscles, and dysfunctional posture all contribute to us getting hurt.

If your muscles and joints are *out of shape*, you become an accident waiting to happen.

- You step off a curb and twist your ankle. That *is* real. But how much did poor alignment, weak muscles in your legs, and lack of flexibility contribute to that happening to you at this time?

- You tore your rotator cuff in your right shoulder when you were playing tennis. But how much did chronically rounded-forward shoulders and lack of flexibility cause that to happen?

- You have back pain. But how much do being overweight and having weak abdominal and low back muscles have to do with that persisting?

- Your doctor says there are signs of arthritis on your X-ray. But how much over the years has lack of activity and loss of flexibility contributed to that?

> Faulty body alignment, weak muscles, and loss of flexibility are, if not the cause, then certainly contributing factors in many of our muscle and joint injuries.

You don't want to get hurt unless you have to. When we injure a knee or ankle or shoulder, particularly as we grow older, things rarely come back to normal. The shoulder, knee, ankle, or hip often doesn't function quite as well as it used to despite the best medical care or surgery.

Injury also causes us to be inactive and for compensations to start rearing their ugly heads. We tilt, we limp, other muscles pick up the slack for their injured brethren. Injury and immobilization themselves cause a global decrease in overall strength and fitness. We don't want all those things to happen.

> We want to prevent injury. Things rarely return completely to normal.

> We have some responsibility to maintain our own muscle and joint health.

What We Need To Do

Here are the four principles of Functional Fitness.

1. We need to stay strong.

We are all often much weaker than we think. The strength of our muscles is what holds us up. There is no substitute for restoring and maintaining muscular strength. Muscle strength supports and protects our joints. We need to strengthen the muscles that support our spines and that allow us to do our everyday activities. And we need to keep it that way.

2. We need to stay flexible.

Inflexibility creeps up at us. Our world—where we can reach and stretch and what we can do—grows smaller. We have to restore and maintain the movement of our joints. Stiffness contributes to joint pain, arthritis, and disability.

3. We need to maintain our posture or body alignment.

Our posture or body alignment is intimately connected with muscle and joint health and function. There is one template where our bodies function most efficiently and economically. When we deviate from that, it causes problems. A slouching, slumping out-of-line body will eventually be a hurting, painful body and one that can no longer do all it is capable of.

4. We need to stay active.

We are animals. We live and thrive on movement. Many of us often curtail or limit movement just at the time in our lives when we need it most.

Stay strong
Stay flexible
Stay aligned
Stay active

After A Certain Age ...

A number of years ago after a particularly long Denver winter where I physically hadn't done much of anything and had gotten totally fat and out of shape, I took my bicycle down from the garage where it had hung suspended all winter. And went for a leisurely ride. But it wasn't.

It was terrible. I huffed. I puffed. I cursed. I sweated. Even little hills that I had previously easily climbed now loomed monstrous. Even with 21 or 27 gears or whatever I had, I still didn't have a gear low enough to climb those hills that day.

The next day a friend of mine who was also in his forties at that time made the following observation. "You know," he said, "after a certain age it's simply easier and makes more sense just to stay in shape." And that phrase stuck with me.

And it's the same thing with our muscle and joint health.

> After a certain age it's easier, smarter, and less expensive in the long run to just do what's necessary to maintain our muscle and joint health.

For most of us that means developing an active exercise program that works for us.

But I Don't Have Time

No one does. But I can understand that. I know what it's like to live a busy life juggling numerous activities and responsibilities around. I know what it's like just to be able to get from one day to the next without having the luxury of exercising.

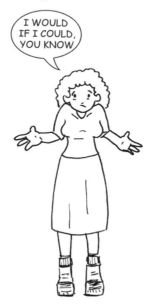

A few simple reminders—

- Your body and your muscle and joint health dramatically affect the quality of your life. If you hurt, a few remedial exercises may get rid of or lessen the pain. If you feel fine now, take action *before* something happens.

- Taking care of your joints makes them *less* of an obtrusion in our lives. And in the long run it may be more costly or expensive in time, money, productivity not to. The best defense is a good offense.

- No one wants to look old before their time. Instead of spending time, effort, and money on cosmetic, superficial solutions, invest your energy in long-term solutions.

Our gradual deterioration in our muscle and joint health is like a river. If you do nothing, you *will* be swept down it in one form or another.

> You have to make maintaining your muscle and joint health a priority.

> It does take time and persistent effort to restore and maintain your strength, flexibility, and alignment. And it's worth it!

You have to see maintaining your muscle and joint health as something with a benefit outweighing the time and effort you invest. For many of us, that possibility doesn't occur until we surface somewhere on the downward spiral. Not to be overly dramatic, but if you don't have time now, you may not have time later.

> Start now.

> Make time.

Certainly, I would prefer that everyone did every exercise in this book and took every bit of my wisdom to heart. Alas, I realize that may be unlikely. But I would like to encourage you at least to *do something*. Start thinking about some of the principles and how they may apply to your life. The exercises in this book are designed like a buffet. There are various exercises you can sample. Try a few. See how you feel. If they help, if they improve the quality of your life, try a few more.

> Do something.

What I Promise

If you read this book, do the exercises, and incorporate some of the new ways of thinking in this book you *will* feel better. You will be able to function in your normal, day-to-day life with more ease and grace. You will want to and be able to physically do more. You will have more energy. You will prevent a great number of problems with your muscles and joints. And if you have problems, many of them may very well go away.

And if all those things aren't enough: Your appearance will improve. You will look younger and feel more vibrant.

> **Change The Way You Think:** You can stay active longer and look younger longer. There are things *you* can do—that no doctor or health care provider can do—that can help prevent muscle and joint pain and disability.

So let's get started. First, let's take a closer look at how the body works and then start stepping off the downward spiral ...

CHAPTER 2

Body Works

*Bones are where they are because
of the position of related myofascial
structures.*

—Ida Rolf

It's Our Muscles That Hold Us Up

That's right—not our bones or skeleton but our muscles. Without our muscles to hold us up, we would be just a pile of bones.

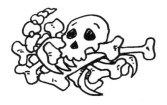

It's our muscles that allow us to do all the things we want to do. And when their strength and flexibility begin to falter we lose our freedom to move.

Our muscles, in great part, also determine the health of our joints. They support, control, and modulate the movement of our joints. Like shock absorbers, they attenuate the compressive forces on our joints. Changes in muscular strength set the stage for joint problems.

> The strength, flexibility, and relative alignment of our muscles determine the overall health of our musculoskeletal system.

Our Muscles Work In Teams

In the olden days two men would saw a log using a long pull saw. One man would push one way while the other relaxed and pulled the other way. It is the same with our muscles. One muscle on one side of the body contracts (pulls) while the opposing muscle on the other side relaxes. This action is what allows us to twist, turn, and make all of the other complicated movements that make up our lives.

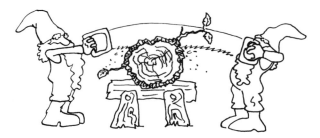

Our whole body is made up of these muscle teams, front to back and side to side. The fancy name for them is agonist-antagonists.

It is only when these teams of muscles work in concert that we have fluid movement. If a muscle one side of the body is stronger than its counterpart on the other side, it leads to imbalance or inequality of labor. It would be as if one of our woodcutters were a big burly fellow and the other a skinny weakling. One side does more of the work and we don't move as well as we should. Physically, we may feel this as a glitch in our stride, or a weakness or sense of "giving way" when we do a certain movement.

Also, if the muscle on one side of the body is chronically tighter or stiffer than its counterpart on the opposite side, we won't be able to bend or stretch as far as we might. It would be akin to one of our woodcutters having short arms or not being able to stretch very far.

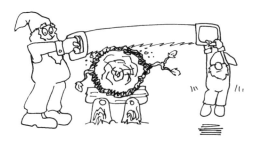

Our body is made up of opposing teams of muscles, and it is their relative strength and flexibility that allows movement.

Neurokinetic Chains Of Motion

Our body is made up of a whole army of these woodcutters. Any simple movement such as getting up off a chair requires the integrated, coordinated action of a whole slew of muscles. And not only do certain muscles on one side have to contract while others relax, but they have to do it in an orderly sequence. An army of woodcutters has to work in concert; certain ones have to pull harder, while others relax, while still others do nothing and then at the exact correct moment pull just slightly. The fancy name for these long connections of muscles sequentially contracting and relaxing in a coordinated fashion is neurokinetic chains of motion. We all inherently recognize this at its best in the grace and fluidity of human movement. It is what keeps us captivated when we see great ballet or figure skating or any great athletic performance.

Sometimes, our optimal sequences may become off (not coordinated). We may not have the strength, flexibility, or alignment to allow what could be called best movement. We may not be using the right muscles in the right way. Or over time, by moving in a sporadic manner, our body may "forget" the optimal way of performing a movement.

Dis-coordinated movement could be considered akin to a string of runway lights coming on one or two at a time, in sporadic bunches, or some not at all.

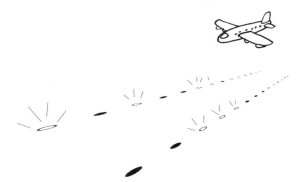

Part of Functional Fitness involves reconfiguring or allowing our bodies to re-remember these optimal sequences of muscle function. The more times and ways you use proper sequences of muscles to perform a movement, the more your body reconfigures itself to make those patterns your home. That's what many of the exercises in this book do.

This is also why it is not necessary for us to go overboard in breaking the body down into various muscle groups and knowing their names and what they do when they contract. It is the sum total of our movement patterns that matters. What we are after is function.

Both Sides

Our bodies are bilaterally symmetrical. The muscles on the right side of our body are mirror images of those on our left. And for proper balance the strength and flexibility of the muscles on the right side of our body should equal that of our left.

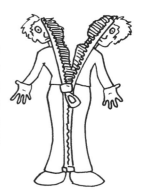

RIGHT = LEFT

Often this isn't the case. One leg or hip may carry more of our weight. Muscles on one side may do more of the work while those on the other side go along for the ride. This causes imbalance of the forces on our joints and on our spine leading to problems. Just as in a relationship, both sides need to be willing and able to do their fair share.

> Our right side should equal our left side in strength and flexibility.

Tensegrity

Buckminster Fuller, the great innovative engineer, created the word "tensegrity" to define the interrelated interdependence of tensile structures. In a tensile structure, each component is suspended and supported by every other component in the structure. Each part of such a structure is in constant interaction with and mutual dependence on each and every other part of such a structure. Like all engineered structures, compression in one area is balanced by tension in another. An example of this is a geodesic ball made up of steel tubes and wires. When one area tightens in response to a stress, another section, by definition, has to relax.

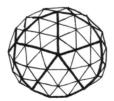

It is the same with our bodies. Our bones are like the tubes of steel and are suspended and supported by a network of muscles, ligaments, and skin. When we move, the connective tissue (muscles, ligaments, and skin) in one part of our body tightens, while another opposing area adjusts and takes up the slack—adjusting and compensating for weight distribution and the effects of gravity. After movement—if our strength and alignment are balanced—we come back to a relatively stress-free position, like our geodesic ball coming back to its normal round shape, in which the stresses are balanced.

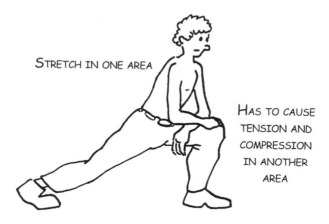

STRETCH IN ONE AREA

HAS TO CAUSE TENSION AND COMPRESSION IN ANOTHER AREA

But if parts of our body are tight or out-of-line on a chronic basis, it not only causes undue tension or compression in that area, but it also *has to* cause undue strain and tension in other parts of the body. Our bodies are integrated wholes. A tight hip joint, for example, while painful in itself, may also affect our low back or knees causing muscle spasm, inflammation, or pain. A rolled-forward shoulder may cause tension in our neck or headaches.

> Our bodies are integrated wholes. Undue stress or tension in one area creates undue stress and tension in other areas.

This is also the reason why the location of a pain may not be its true source. You may be hurting in your shoulder, but it may be a twist or tilt in your hips that is causing increased tension to be transmitted to your shoulder. The shoulder is simply where it is felt. Often, only by remedying the hip problem will the shoulder problem be solved. Your knees may hurt, but it may be weakness of your leg muscles that allows the compressive forces of your weight to be felt in your knees.

> The location of a pain is often not its true source.

A tilted or out-of-line joint in one part of the body can cause pain or problems virtually *anywhere* in the body. For example, a tilted hip can cause pain not only in the hip or buttocks, but also in the knee, ankle, foot, or even up into the low back or into the shoulders. Because our muscles form a cascade that interconnects our entire body, the pain may be felt on the side of the mal-alignment or even on the other side.

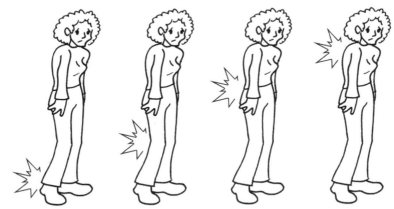

Compensation And Improvisation

Our bodies are great improvisers. They are expert at making do with what's available. They have to be. If every time we cut ourselves or bruised an arm or leg we were knocked totally out of commission, we wouldn't have lasted long as a species. If we sprain an ankle, our body figures out a method of circumventing the use of the injured ankle allowing a chance for the injured area to heal. In road construction the cars are detoured around the section of road being repaired. In the same way, the body rests the injured area and enlists other muscles not usually used for that job to pitch in and help out.

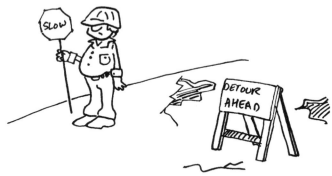

It says, "Hey, this area hurts over here so you muscles over there have to help out while this area rests." And other muscles pitch in allowing us to walk, perhaps in a slightly awkward manner but nonetheless getting the job done.

In effect, our bodies jerry-rig a solution if at all possible by using our hips, knees, and shoulders in ways they aren't generally accustomed to, like swinging them out to the side, holding one arm up for balance like an outrigger, or carrying most of our weight on one side and getting by.

A problem arises when muscles that aren't supposed to be doing a certain job end up being permanently assigned to that position, such as when we never regain strength after an injury.

We also compensate and improvise in smaller ways on a day-to-day basis. When we don't use certain muscles for long stretches of time, they become weak. If we predominately sit for much of our day, certain muscles become weak. Then when those weak muscles are called upon to do their job, they aren't up to it. Other muscles take up the slack. We walk with muscles that aren't designed for walking. We lift using muscles not designed for lifting. Again, we aren't aware of this; it sneaks up on us. At first this compensation works. But over time it invariably leads to problems.

Our body compensates and improvises as long as it can. But eventually a muscle that is doing its own job *and someone else's job* has enough and screams, "I can't do it anymore!" It begins to hurt or goes into spasm. Eventually a joint that is doing most of the work for both sides of the body throws in the towel. It becomes inflamed and sits down on the job.

Compensation or improvisation in one area of the body also leads to compensation and improvisation in other areas. When one area that is working overtime can do it no longer, it falls to the wayside, and another area starts to take up the slack. Like a faltering chain of command, when the muscles in our hip can no longer carry our weight, the weight is transferred to our back muscles. When our back muscles cry out and are no longer up to the job, perhaps we tilt our hips a little when we walk to enlist another muscle group. And on it goes.

> Compensation and improvisation in one area beget further compensation and improvisation in other areas.

We become the sum total of all our compensations and improvisations. And what started off as a simple problem (with often a simple solution) has now become a convoluted complex problem. If our body could talk, it might go something like this—

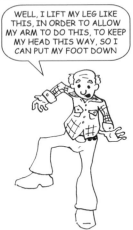

WELL, I LIFT MY LEG LIKE THIS, IN ORDER TO ALLOW MY ARM TO DO THIS, TO KEEP MY HEAD THIS WAY, SO I CAN PUT MY FOOT DOWN

> We want to avoid compensations. We want every part of our body to be doing its appropriate job.

In medicine, sometimes a person comes to a doctor's office with literally a whole grocery bag full of medications. There are pills to treat an original problem, and then there are pills to treat the side effects of those pills. Then there are pills prescribed by another doctor for other problems. Then there are pills to counteract the interactions of those pills with the first pills.

Sometimes the best solution is to stop everything and start over. It is the same with our muscles and joints. Sometimes rather than trying to dissect every pain and disability, it makes more sense to simply start over and just focus on getting all our muscles strong, flexible, and aligned.

> With regard to musculoskeletal health, the only long-term solution is to get all our muscles strong enough, flexible enough, and aligned so that they all consistently do the jobs they are intended to do.

Alignment

In human beings (as in any segmented biological structure), movement is determined by joints.

—Ida Rolf

Joints occur where two bones meet. Joints allow us to move. Ligaments are the fibrous bands that hold joints together. But it is the relative strength and alignment of our muscles that determine the forces placed on our joints. If the muscle on one side of a joint is too tight while its counterpart is too loose, there is a slight cocking of a joint, a tilt.

This causes increased force on one side of the joint as opposed to the other. This causes the ligaments that support the joint on one side to be stretched (increased tension) as opposed to the other side. This, in turn, puts our joint at risk for injury and for increased wear and tear.

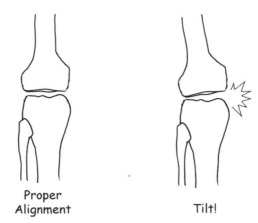

Proper
Alignment   Tilt!

The strength of muscles surrounding a joint also provides *lift* to a joint. Strong muscles keep our joints from collapsing down on themselves and bone from forcibly colliding with and rubbing against bone. Like shock absorbers, they attenuate the compressive forces placed on our joints.

The relative strength and flexibility of our muscles also determine the overall alignment of our bodies—our posture. Imagine not just one joint being slightly tilted but multiple joints being tilted. Our posture is the composite of all our tilted joints. It is the sum total of some muscles being too tight, some muscles being overly strong, and some muscles being weak that determines our overall positioning in space.

Proper alignment or posture is so important to muscle and joint health that several chapters in this book are devoted exclusively to it.

Gravity

We may think of gravity as something that allows apples to fall from trees or as something the shuttle craft has to overcome to leave the earth's atmosphere. But gravity also plays an important role in our musculoskeletal system. Gravity is a vertical vector force pushing down on our bodies from above. And until the day we die, we carry on a constant war with this force called gravity.

> Left to its devices gravity conspires to shorten us,
> thicken us, and make us closer to the ground.

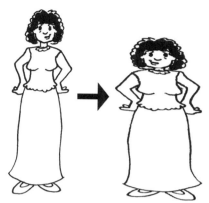

What holds us up against the constant flow of gravity? Our muscles. We each carry on our own individual battle with gravity throughout our lives, and our individual postures are, in part, our individual solutions to dealing with this problem.

The more vertically aligned and upright we are, the more gravity flows off us much the way water flows off a vertical statue or building. When we are chronically hunched over, slouched, or off balance, gravity forms eddies around our protruding parts.

When our alignment is off, it takes additional energy to hold ourselves up against gravity. The muscles required to hold us up in unnatural postures become tired and fatigued and often contribute to us slouching even more.

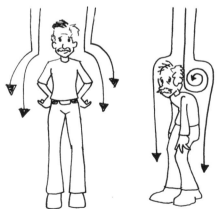

Function Creates Form

*The form of the human body is the
result of the sum of its everyday
movements.*

—Bess Mensendick[1]

Our bodies function the way they do because of the demands placed on us over millions of years of evolution. And the smaller variations in our form and function—fat, thin, tilted, weak, strong—represent the demands, or lack thereof, placed on us on a daily, weekly, monthly, and yearly basis.

> Our individual variations—the way our bodies look and function—are a direct result of what we are doing or not doing.

All world-class breaststrokers look almost alike. All Olympic gymnasts have virtually identical bodies. In any sport, the highest level of performance requires, demands, and creates a certain body form and functional ability.

It's the same with the rest of us. The reason so many people's postures look alike—unfortunately, often slouched or hunched over—is because they have similar demands or lack of demands placed on them. It is also the reason so many of us are prone to the same muscle and joint ailments and disabilities. What we do or don't do determines our form and our function and what we will be able to do in the future.

> Our bodies are created and re-created on a daily basis by what we do or don't do.

> **Change The Way You Think:** Muscle strength, flexibility, and alignment in great part, determine our muscle and joint health. Our bodies are integrated wholes. Stress, tension, or mal-alignment in one area has to be transmitted or felt in other areas. The location of a pain is often not its source. Until we die, we fight a war against gravity. Our form and function is determined by what we do or don't do.

In the next chapter, we'll take a closer look at the aging process—at what we're up against ...

Suggested Resources

Rolfing, Reestablishing the Natural Alignment and Structural Integration of the Human Body for Vitality and Well-Being, Ida Rolf, PhD, Healing Arts Press, 1989. Although this book is about Rolfing, a form of deep mysofascial bodywork, it is also one of the better books on functional anatomy and includes many original insights into our body's form and function.

---

1 Author of *It's Up to You,* 1931—a very forward-thinking woman on exercise and the importance of posture.

CHAPTER 3

Aging

> But at my back I always hear
> Times's winged chariot
> Hurrying near.
>
> —Andrew Marvel

The facts on aging are not in our favor. As if you weren't already aware of it, there *are* incontrovertible changes in our bodies with aging. Not only do our hearts, lungs, livers, and spleens undergo age-related changes, but so do our muscles and joints. They *don't* work as efficiently as they used to, and they don't work up to the same standards as when we were twenty or thirty or even forty or fifty.

It should be a sobering fact that musculoskeletal disability *is* the most common cause of chronic disability in people sixty-five or older. But a premise of this book is that there are things we do that contribute to or cause some of the muscle and joint changes commonly attributed to aging, and there are things we can do to attenuate or put off some of the effects of these changes.

> We have the ability to forestall many of the changes we commonly associate with aging with regard to our muscle and joint systems.

But here are a few of the things we are up against …

Bone Loss

We lose bone as we age. Our bones get weaker and more susceptible to collapse and fracture. Peak bone mass occurs between the ages of twenty and thirty followed by a gradual but progressive loss in bone mass in both sexes.

Women have lower peak bone mass to begin with than men. In women, bone loss occurs at a rate of 0.75–1%/year beginning at age 30 to 35. Following menopause there is period of rapid bone loss (2–3 %/year) that lasts for about ten years, which is superimposed on the age-related bone loss in all individuals. At this rate women can lose 30% bone mineral mass by age seventy.

Bone loss occurs earlier in the spine than in the limbs. Also, our spinal discs lose water content with aging. These two factors contribute to a loss of height of about 2 cm/decade between the ages of sixty and eighty.

These bone-loss changes put women in particular at risk for osteoporosis, a disease characterized by decreased bone mass, enhanced bone fragility, and an increased risk of fractures. The real danger of osteoporosis is this risk of fractures. If you do fall, you are more likely to break something. Unfortunately, it is often a hip that is fractured that causes both significant mortality and disability in the older individual.

What can you do about these bone-loss changes?

Although osteoporosis does occur in men, women in particular should be routinely evaluated by their physicians for their risk of osteoporosis with appropriate diagnostic tests and medical treatment (most often medications) when indicated. All women should take supplemental calcium as indicated.

Stay strong. Strengthening exercises in women (weight lifting for example) have been shown to slow down or at least limit bone loss. Bones respond to getting strong. The pulling on the bone actually causes new bone to be laid down and the redistribution of internal bony architecture in alignment with the new forces. By staying strong you also reduce your risk of falling. If you are about to fall, you are more apt to catch yourself. You have a functional reserve of strength available for emergency situations. If you do fall, you have the strength to break your fall, thereby potentially avoiding serious injury.

As an aside, since peak bone mass growth occurs in the teens, it is critically important that young girls in particular get adequate calcium, vitamin D *and* exercise. The bone mass developed in the teen years serves as a bone repository for the rest of your life. The more bone mineral mass you can lay down at that time, the more you have to draw on as you age.

Muscle Changes

Physiologically we lose muscle strength with aging. Muscle strength peaks at around age thirty, remains relatively constant to age fifty, and then declines.

With aging if we do nothing, we lose 5 to 7 pounds of muscle every decade. Our muscle body mass in great part determines our metabolism. Decrease in muscle mass causes a reduction in our resting metabolic at a rate of 2 to 5% per decade. This makes it easy to become overweight. Staying strong (Chapter 7) helps to limit this loss of muscle and increases our resting metabolic rate and our caloric requirements, thereby reducing the likelihood of fat accumulation.

Loss of muscle strength leads to limitation in daily activities, loss of independence, arthritis and joint problems, and an increased risk of falls and fractures.

As we grow older, we also lose "fast-twitch" muscle fibers. These are responsible for quick movements and in part determine our reaction time. This is one reason older individuals are more prone to falls—they can't react quickly enough to catch themselves.

As we age, our muscles take a longer time to repair themselves and to recover after exercise. After strenuous exercise, our bodies don't bounce back quite as quickly. If we are hurt or immobilized, it takes longer to regain our lost strength.

However, although some of our loss of strength with aging is biologically mandated, all of it is not. Relative inactivity and disuse of muscles compound our problems.

Any muscle when not used loses strength. When a muscle is immobilized, for example, when a leg is placed in plaster cast for several weeks, it rapidly loses strength. One recent study reports a 13% decrease in lower extremity strength in healthy subjects who underwent only ten days of non-weight-bearing activity. Immobilization causes atrophy of muscle tissue and loss of sarcomeres (the contractile building blocks of muscle). And it often takes *years* to fully recover this strength.

When immobilized or not used, muscles also lose extensibility. On a microscopic level, muscles act like zippers; they unzip when they stretch and zip together when they contract. If left shortened for long periods of time, they can lose some of their zippering ability, causing us to lose some of the zip in our step.

> With immobilization, we lose muscle strength and extensibility at an astounding rate, and it takes a long time to recover.

You already know this if you have ever been sick or immobilized for an extended period of time. It takes a long time to get your strength back.

But disuse or inactivity are also forms of immobilization. When we don't use a muscle or only use it on rare occasions, the same biological changes occur. With lack of use or minimal use, muscle groups also microscopically lose sarcomeres, along with their zipping and unzipping ability.

> The effects of disuse on muscles are similar to the effects of immobilization.

However, one of the miracles of the human body, and of muscle in particular, is its resiliency. We have the ability to regain muscle strength. And there isn't some magic age at which we lose the ability to create stronger muscles. In one study, patients in their eighties and nineties increased quadriceps strength 175% over a 12-week period, producing functional improvement in such things as getting out of chairs and going up steps. It's never too late. Until the day we die, our muscles respond to demand. When we consistently place a demand on our muscles greater than what they are used to, they *will* grow stronger (more on this in Chapter 7).

You can't completely defeat the natural changes in muscles with aging but you can hold many of them at bay.

> Get strong and stay strong.

Tendons, Ligaments, And Cartilage

Tendons are the fibrous connective tissue at the tail end of muscles that attach them to bone. Ligaments are the fibrous connective tissue that surround and stabilize our joints. Ligaments act like guy wires reacting to tensile force by becoming taut. In this way they protect and control joint movement.

With aging, both tendons and ligaments lose water content and become less able to withstand tensile loads. In effect, this means ligaments are neither as strong nor as flexible and can't stabilize joints as well. If not used, tendons reform themselves, becoming shorter and thicker.

Cartilage is the Teflon-like lining in joints. It allows our joints to glide effortlessly—and hopefully painlessly—through their ranges of motion. With aging, cartilage also loses water content and becomes less efficient at buffering joint movement. All types of arthritis involve a breakdown or inflammation of cartilage; some of it is age-related. This is discussed in more detail in Chapter 11.

Weight

> *To lengthen thy Life,*
> *lessen thy Meals.*
>
> —Benjamin Franklin
> *Poor Richard's Almanack*

With aging, our metabolism changes, and for most of us this means it becomes easier to gain weight, harder to lose it, and harder to keep it off. Much of this is mediated by the hormonal changes associated with aging. Just as excessive weight is a risk factor for other disease (hypertension, diabetes, heart disease), excessive weight also places our musculoskeletal system at risk. Excess weight increases the loading forces on all our joints, and hence, the potential for wear and tear and injury to them.

Because of body mechanics, increases in weight *exponentially* increase the force on many of our key load-bearing joints, notably our knees, hips, and backs. The effects of any alteration in our alignment are magnified. Any disparities in our posture will also have a tendency to be made that much more permanent.

Excessive weight accelerates wear and tear on our joints, and hence has the potential to subtract years from the effective lives of our joints.

> Excessive weight increases the loads carried by our joints and multiplies the effects of any mal-alignment we may have. Thus, it increases the likelihood for musculoskeletal pain and disability.

Too much weight also makes us less likely to be active; it simply takes too much effort. Our weight becomes the limiting factor in what we can or cannot do.

> It takes more effort to do things when we weigh too much, and hence we become less active.

But it also affects us in smaller ways. We become less likely to walk a short distance, less likely to bend down, less likely to do a whole host of small physical activities that make up our daily life. And we are more likely to fall.

The combined effects of excess weight make us more prone to the downward spiral. Increased weight leads to relative inactivity. Relative inactivity leads to more muscle weakness and stiffness. Muscle stiffness and weakness compromise our posture and alignment. Muscle weakness, stiffness, and mal-alignment set the stage for joint and muscle pain and disability. And because we are less active and because we hurt, we often gain even more weight.

> Lose weight and keep it off.

The Hip Bone's Connected To The ... Spleen

Our bodies are integrated wholes. The functioning of our hearts, lungs, livers, and spleens affects the health of our muscles and joints. Our heart's ability to pump blood, our lungs ability to bring in oxygen, the functioning of our digestive tract, the pumping of lymph—all these things and more affect the health of our muscles and joints.

With aging, any compromise in any of our systems has the potential to make us prone to the downward spiral in muscle and joint health.

> The health of our bodies as a whole affects the health of our muscles and joints. The health of our muscles and joints affects the health of our bodies as a whole.

That's why maintaining overall health remains part of an effective muscle and joint longevity plan.

What Makes Us Look Old Anyway?

The idea is to die young as late as possible.

—Ashley Montagu

Sure, it shows in our face, skin, and hair. And a huge industry has emerged to alleviate or buffer some of these changes that accompany aging—replete with Botox, hair color, wrinkle-removing creams, cosmetic surgery and a host of other treatments. But aging also shows in our posture and in the way we move. Or to be more accurate, in the way we don't move.

Older people (whatever age you pick for that) generally move slower and in a more limited, restricted manner. They can't reach as far up, down, or to the sides. They hoist themselves up and down out of chairs. Therefore, rather than focusing solely on the more superficial aspects of aging (skin and hair), if we are indeed interested in preserving our relative youth, it might make more sense to make sure we are doing all we can to preserve our movement potential.

Most of the chapters that follow contain exercise recommendations. The exercises are listed in mini-menus. That way, once you have mastered the exercises, you can refer to one page of the book or make copies of the appropriate pages. All of the exercises in this book are listed in one chapter, Chapter 13. Where exercises are recommended in the text, a thumbnail picture of the exercise is shown along with the page number where a detailed description of the exercise can be found.

Make sure to read the beginning of Chapter 13 before doing any of the exercises. And the first few times you do an exercise, refer back to the detailed instructions for that exercise. Some of the exercises may seem like ones you have done before, but there are often key differences that make them more effective.

> Detailed instructions for all exercises are given in Chapter 13.

You don't want to look old before your time. Here are some key ways older people move, what they mean, and a few simple starter exercises you can do to help start remedying the problem.

Function Exercises

Trouble Getting Up From Sitting

Symptom: Having to push off on your legs or the arms of the chair every time you get up.

What It Means: Weakness of leg muscles often quadriceps muscle.

Imaginary Chair
Page 174

Wall Bench
Page 188

Squats
Page 182

Difficulty Reaching or Stretching Up Above Your Head

Symptom: Difficulty lifting one or both arms straight up directly above your head; limited range of motion at the shoulder; rounded, rolled forward shoulders.

What It Means: Tightness of muscles in the front of chest and surrounding shoulders; weakness of muscles in upper back and between shoulder blades.

Arm Circles
Page 163

Elbow Curls
Page 170

Overhead Stretch
Page 179

Face the Wall
Page 171

Face Plant
Page 170

Trouble Bending Down and Reaching for Things

Symptom: Weakness or a sense that your legs will give way when we you have to bend down and stretch to reach something.

What It Means: Weakness and stiffness of quadriceps and hamstrings

Warrior II
Page 188

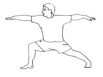

Reaching Down
Under
Page 180

Deep Squat
Page 169

Trouble Twisting

Symptom: Having to get up and turn your whole body to see behind you; trouble checking blind spot when driving.

What It Means: Stiffness and tightness of muscles and connective tissue surrounding shoulders, pelvis, and flanks.

Chair Twist
Page 166

Floor Twist
Page 172

Standing Bent-Knee
Chair Twist
Page 183

Standing Side
Stretch
Page 184

Lying Side
Stretch
Page 178

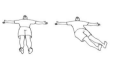

Triangle
Page 187

Trouble Tying Shoes

Symptom: Okay, you wear loafers or sandals. But for many people as they grow older, a real Catch-22 develops—you can't bend enough to reach down where shoe and foot are and your hip can't bend enough to get your foot up on your thigh. Here are a few exercises to improve flexibility for both methods: #1—bringing you down to your shoe and #2—bringing the shoe up to you.

What It Means: Inflexibility of back muscles and tightness of hips.

Child's Pose
on Chair
Page 167

Child's Pose
Page 166

Couch Stretch
Page 168

Forward Bend
at Wall
Page 172

Crossover
Hip Stretch
Page 168

Floor Twist
Page 172

Leg Flop
Page 175

Pigeon
Page 179

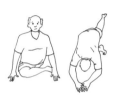

One final word—I would be remiss if I didn't mention that with aging, for whatever reasons, it *does* seem to take more effort to start or restart an exercise program. It *does* take more effort to get out there and do something. The gains and results do seem to come slower. Accept that, but remember that you are doing something for yourself that will bear results for many years to come.

Change The Way You Think: There are incontrovertible changes that occur in muscles and joints with aging. But there are things we can do to attenuate their effect on us. Part of looking old is how we move.

Next, let's take a closer look at a key factor in our muscle and joint health and function—our posture or body alignment ...

CHAPTER 4

The Importance Of Posture

*A weight-bearing joint will be mechanically
balanced and in equilibrium only if the gravity
line of the mass it supports falls exactly
through the axis of rotation.*

—Daniels, *Therapeutic Exercise*

Posture—the word itself sounds old-fashioned. Like something best relegated to earlier times when Victorian women carried books around on their heads or sat upright in stiff-backed chairs during long afternoon teas.

But posture is more relevant now than ever and plays a key role in preserving and maintaining our muscle and joint health, particularly as we grow older. If you just look around, more and more people are becoming more and more crooked, slouched, and just generally out of line and at earlier and earlier ages.

What we are really talking about when we say posture is our body's alignment, both the alignment of our body as a whole and the alignment of individual joints. Alterations in our posture directly influence what we can or cannot comfortably do and can cause much of the muscle and joint aches, pains, and disability as we grow older. Our posture also affects how we look. People with poor posture look old before their time.

Correct posture should not be some stiff, soldier-like position you assume or put yourself into. It is not about "holding ourselves there." Correct posture can be described as a position of equipoise. It is where our bodies should naturally and gracefully come back to after all our reaching, stretching, lifting, and other forays into the world of movement. Like coming home at the end of the day.

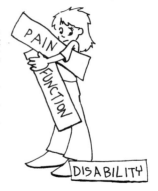

> Correct posture is not forced. It should be where we naturally reside.

The Body As A Machine

Our bodies are like machines, and like any machine they operate best when things are properly aligned. We wouldn't expect a machine in a factory to operate optimally if the gears weren't correctly aligned or if the weight wasn't correctly balanced along a centerline; it is the same way with our bodies.

Our bodies are designed to have a certain alignment for optimal functioning. When we are tilted, hunched over, or leaning, the vertical axis of our body is altered. Our weight is carried disproportionately more on one side than the other, or our weight is concentrated excessively on one joint, a hip for example, or one area of our back. Some muscles work overtime holding us up while others skate by doing almost nothing. The load and work schedule aren't equally distributed.

Each of our individual muscles is also designed to pull in a specific direction. When things are crooked or off-center, muscles don't pull in the optimal direction they were designed to. They don't work as efficiently as they might. It is akin to trying to pull or pry up something with the fulcrum in the wrong position. Over time it leads to things breaking down.

Weight being carried more on one side - some muscles doing more of the work.

> When our posture is off—when our body is not properly aligned—the machine doesn't work as well as it should.

The articular surfaces of our joints are also designed for our weight to be carried with a specific alignment. Ideally, for any given joint, the weight it carries should be carried through the central axis of the joint and equally distributed throughout the entire joint surface.

When a joint is tilted or off-center, there are increased compressive forces and, consequently, increased wear and tear on one side of the joint as opposed to the other. There is also a disproportionate amount of tension on the ligaments on one side of the joint as opposed to the other. An out-of-line joint is one that is more likely to be injured.

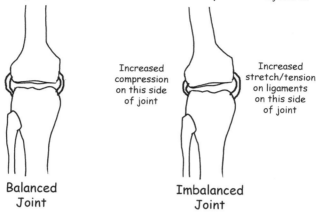

Increased compression on this side of joint

Increased stretch/tension on ligaments on this side of joint

Balanced Joint

Imbalanced Joint

> Deviation from proper alignment produces asymmetrical forces on our joints.

Optimal Alignment

Anatomists, orthopedists, sports medicine specialists, chiropractors, and biomechanical engineers all come to the same conclusions on how our bodies should be aligned for optimal function—on how our body was *designed* to function.

> The more we deviate from optimal posture, the more likely we are to have problems with our muscles and joints.

Here is a brief overview of this optimal alignment.

Our major joints—shoulders, hips, knees, and ankles—should be vertically aligned. Look at the picture below. From the front, if we draw a vertical line down from our shoulder joint area, ideally it should intersect our hip, knee, and ankle joints. In a gravity-constrained world, vertical alignment produces the least amount of stress and strain on component parts.

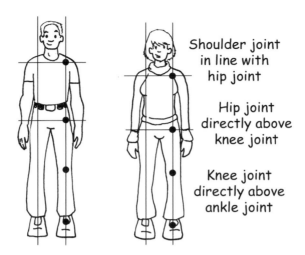

Shoulder joint
in line with
hip joint

Hip joint
directly above
knee joint

Knee joint
directly above
ankle joint

One hip, knee, ankle, or shoulder shouldn't be higher or lower or more out to the side than its counterpart on the other side. Many of us have one or more parts that are either tilted or higher or lower than their compadres on the other side.

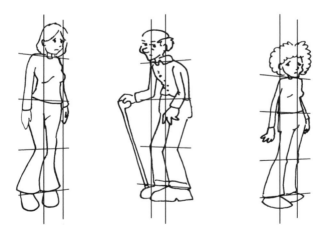

Our major joints should also line up when seen from the side. Ideally, from the side a vertical line should intersect our ankle, knee, hip, shoulder, and ear. Our body as a whole also shouldn't be leaning or falling forward or backward.

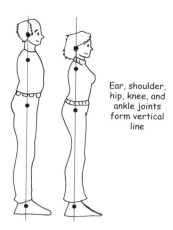

Ear, shoulder, hip, knee, and ankle joints form vertical line

Again, many of us have one or more parts that are forward or behind this vertical plumb line.

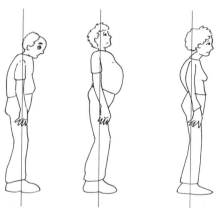

All of our major joints should line up.

Our body works best when it is vertically aligned.

The major bones in our lower extremities—thighs, legs, ankles, and feet—should ideally point straight ahead. Our lower extremity joints are all basically hinge joints in the frontal plane, and for forward motion we want the hinges to be opening and closing in the forward direction. This means, for example, that one or both knees shouldn't point out to the side or inward. Our feet in particular should point straight ahead or close to it, and be neither turned inward nor splayed way out to the side like a duck (more on this in Chapter 6).

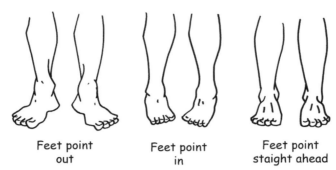

Feet point
out

Feet point
in

Feet point
staight ahead

Our spines are designed to carry our weight with three gentle curves somewhat like an "S".

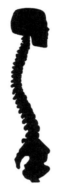

Too much or too little curve in our upper or lower back causes our weight to be carried forward or behind our central axis. It also causes a disproportionate amount of our weight to be carried by one part of our spine (often our lower back) rather than being equally distributed throughout our entire spine.

> Our spine is designed to carry our weight with a gentle, S-shaped curve.

Our pelvis, the linchpin of our body's alignment, is linked to the curves in our back and is designed to be aligned horizontally and not tilted too far forward or backward. The illustrations are somewhat exaggerated; the tilt need not be as dramatic to have a decided effect on our alignment.

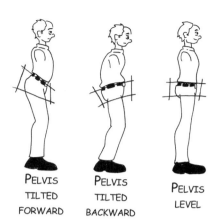

PELVIS
TILTED
FORWARD

PELVIS
TILTED
BACKWARD

PELVIS
LEVEL

A pelvis that is tilted too far forward causes the curve in our low back to be *increased* or exaggerated and alters our center of gravity. Our belly tends to spill forward and we often bring our shoulders back to compensate to keep from falling forward.

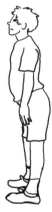

A pelvis that is tilted or slumped backward is a little harder to see. From the side, it appears as if the person is almost sitting or slouched backward even while standing. The curve in the low back is *decreased* or completely gone. Often the shoulders are hunched and rolled forward.

A lifestyle where we sit a lot and slouch in chairs makes us particularly prone to a backward-tilted pelvis.

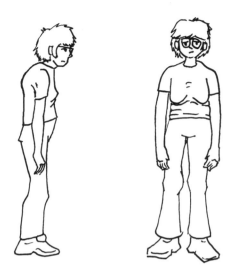

> Our pelvis is designed to be aligned horizontally and neither tilted too far forward nor backward.

Because the pelvis is so important to our alignment, it will be discussed in more detail in the next chapter.

Our shoulders work best when they are back. Think of classic Greek or Roman sculpture. The shoulders are back and the chest is opened and expanded. Unfortunately, rolled-forward, rounded shoulders are very common. The alignment of our pelvis and the curves in our low back in great part determine the positioning of our shoulders. Weak muscles in our backs and around our pelvis often contribute to our upper backs hunching forward and our shoulders rounding forward. Altered shoulder positioning can contribute not only to shoulder problems but also to problems with our elbows, wrists, and hands (see box below).

Our shoulders should also be level, that is, one shouldn't be higher, lower, or more forward than the other.

Rounded Shoulders

Particularly as we grow older, there is often a tendency for our shoulders to roll forward and our upper back to become more hunched. Along with this, our head often juts forward.

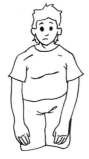 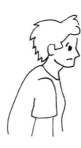 If our shoulders and upper back are rounded too far forward, we lose *function*. We become unable to reach as far over our heads or behind us.

Try this. Sit up straight and purposely roll your shoulders forward so that the backs of your hands point straight ahead. Now keeping your shoulders in that position, try to reach overhead. You can't reach very far. It's only when our shoulders are back in their proper position that we have full range of motion.

If our shoulders and upper back are rounded too far forward, it contributes to *pain and disability*. There is increased tension and strain in the muscles behind our necks and shoulders. A chronic, collapsed position constricts full expansion of our chest and limits our breathing, and can potentially put pressure on the nerves and blood vessels that run beneath our arms.

Our heads are heavy—about 10 to 15 pounds, like a bowling ball. It takes considerable muscular strain to hold our heavy head out at an angle in the gravitational jet stream. Is it surprising we have headaches, neck and back pain?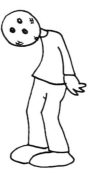

And finally, our posture affects our *appearance*. Rolled-forward shoulders and a hunched upper back make us look old and ineffectual before our time.

The Effects Of Bad Posture

When our posture or alignment gets off, it no longer feels good to do things. The machine doesn't work the way it should, and at some intuitive level we all sense this.

Physically, we become reluctant to be as active. We resist doing as many physical activities as we might. And we often don't know why—it just doesn't feel right or fun or comfortable anymore. "Don't wanna." "Don't feel like it." "Got other things I gotta do."

In our minds we make a microsecond assessment of what a physical activity might entail. We check with how our body feels, and enter a yea or nay vote on the activity. It is often disparities in our posture or alignment that contribute to a disinclination to be active.

> When our posture is off, we naturally don't want to do as much. It becomes harder, and it's simply no fun.

Any curtailment of activity, particularly as we grow older, sets the stage for further curtailment of activity. The downward spiral again—

We aren't as active as we used to be.
We lose muscle strength.
Our alignment gets worse.
We are even more reluctant to be active.
We lose more muscle strength.
We become stiffer.
We hurt.
We get injured.
We are less active.

> Alterations in our posture or alignment contribute to a cascade of effects, which further limit and compromise our muscle and joint function.

Remember, we want to limit any chinks in our musculoskeletal armor that may make us more prone to the downward spiral. Compromise in our posture is one of these.

Are there people out there with tilted pelvises, the wrong curves in their backs, and with their joints lined up asunder who seem to function without any problems? Sure there are. But for most of us—and this includes you and me—the more we deviate from correct alignment, the more prone we are to pain, injury, disability, and overall loss of function.

When our posture is off, we also look old before our time. We look faltering. People with more upright posture are perceived as more confident, happy, and in control of their lives. Good posture signals health and confidence. Slouching signals weakness and self-doubt.

> Those with more erect posture are seen as younger and more vibrant.

And we look thinner. That's right, even without losing weight. Yes, it could be an ad for a miracle cure. Here's how it works. As we grow older, many of us lose the supporting tone in our muscles, primarily the muscles in our backs and abdomen. We lose the supporting muscular strength in our spines. Our pelvis begins to tilt forward or backward. We begin to collapse down on ourselves; our abdomens bulge outward. Some of that pouch around our midsections is due to our sagging postures. Stand up straight and see how much of your belly disappears. We don't have to "hold it in."

Women Only:
Nothing Destroys A Good Outfit More Than Bad Posture

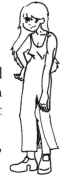

You've finally bought the outfit or suit you've dreamed about. It's the perfect size and color. And it was even marked down 50%. But when you put it on at home, it doesn't look quite right.

Why? Bad posture. Slumping rounded shoulders, sagging back, paunch in the belly.

Correcting your posture can help.

Why Do Our Postures Vary?

Simply put, we each created our own individual postures by what we did in the past, and we each re-create our posture by what we are doing and not doing now.

If we don't move enough in certain ways, some muscles become stiff, tight, and less flexible. If we sit a lot at our jobs, certain sitting muscles (yes, there are sitting muscles) become strong, and other muscles become somewhat ...flabby. It is this interplay of muscle strength, weakness, stiffness, and looseness that holds each of us in our individual postures. We are each a perfect composite of all these varying forces. It is what makes us able to say at a distance, "There's Bob," or "Here comes Sally."

And it is the sum total of our daily demands (or lack thereof) that *perpetuates* each of our individual postures. It is the muscles we are using or not using. It is the muscles that are being stretched or not being stretched. And over time, not just muscles, but ligaments, skin, fascia, other connective tissue, and even bone begin to conform and adjust to our altered positions contributing to our becoming more "fixed" in our characteristic posture.

> The combination of certain muscles being weak, certain muscles being strong, and certain muscles being tight is what holds each of us in our individual posture.

Can injuries cause alterations in our posture? Sure they can. But more often than not, it is not the injury itself, but the fact that we never fully recovered and regained correct alignment and muscle use *after the injury* that causes the persistence of an altered posture. Our bones and ligaments may have healed, but our compensation for the injury may have persisted.

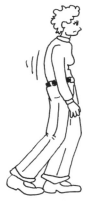

CERTAIN MUSCLES BEING TIGHT AND CERTAIN MUSCLES BEING WEAK HOLD EACH OF US IN OUR INDIVIDUAL POSTURES

Quirks

Whatever little quirks in our alignment we may have now often become deeper and more pronounced as we grow older. A person with a little slump looks more slumped the next time we see them. Why? Because by continuing to use the same muscles, which created the quirks in our posture to begin with, we tend to perpetuate the idiosyncrasies of our own individual posture.

> By continuing to use the same muscles in the same ways, we perpetuate our individual posture, and over time our idiosyncrasies become more pronounced.

If we aren't careful, shoulders that are slightly slumped forward now slump forward even more as we grow older. If we favor one hip now, over time we will tend to favor that hip even more.

In effect, with time we become more ingrained versions of ourselves—posture-wise. There's an old maxim in self-help circles: If you keep doing what you've always done, you'll keep getting what you've always got. It's the same with our bodies.

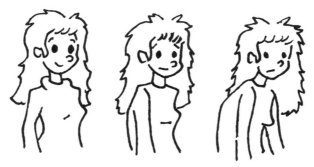

> If you keep giving your body the same stimulus and using the same muscles you've always used, your posture will remain the same and you'll keep looking the way you've always looked.

To change things, you have to do something different. Just as with our relationships, finances, or anything else that may have gotten into a rut, it's the same with our muscle and joints. We have to provide new direction and stimulus to change. Muscle-wise, we have to do things we aren't doing now.

> To change your posture, you have to give your body different stimuli. You have to stretch muscles that are tight, strengthen the muscles that are weak, and use muscles that you may not be using.

"Okay, Enough Already, I'll Pull My Shoulders Back And Sit Up Straight ..."

Won't work. But you already know that. After a few seconds, your body returns to its "normal" position. Tight muscles are like strong rubber bands. Weak muscles can't hold out against them, and the tight, strong muscles pull us back into our normal position.

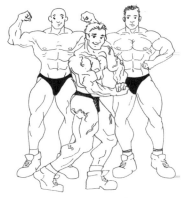

FORGET IT!
YOU CAN'T HOLD
OUT AGAINST US!

That's why it takes a more concerted effort to change our posture. We need to systematically stretch the muscles that are tight and strengthen the muscles that are weak. Often big, tight muscles in one area of our body—most often our pelvis—hold us captive in our posture. Until we get them to loosen up and relinquish their control, our bodies will tend to spring back to their old positions. This takes time.

> To change our posture, we need to stretch the
> muscles that are tight, strengthen the muscles that
> are weak, and align ourselves in new and hopefully
> more optimal positioning.

We have to get muscles that may not have been doing their job to get back to work. We have to retrain our bodies to use the right muscles to hold us up in the right places.

An entire chapter (Chapter 9) is devoted to exercises that help restore and preserve our posture and alignment.

A Small Change Can Make A Big Difference

While achieving some mythical perfect posture may be a noble goal for some, for many of us even just a small correction or improvement in our posture can make a difference. A small change in our posture can make a big difference, both now and in the years to come. Correcting or improving your posture *even slightly* may be enough to take pressure off a joint, to redistribute forces that are grinding away at a bone surface, and to get rid of a pain that has been nagging you for years. A small change in your posture may be enough to give a muscle that has been working overtime for years a chance to recover.

A small change in your posture now may prevent any quirks in your posture from becoming more pronounced.

A small improvement in your posture may allow you to keep doing activities you might otherwise be forced to give up, and to keep you looking younger longer.

Improving our posture now can prevent pain or disability in the future and keep you functional longer in the years to come.

> A small improvement in your posture can make a big
> difference.

One final thought—if all else fails, you are perfectly welcome to carry this book around on your head.

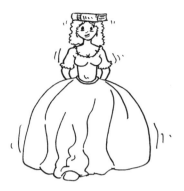

> **Change The Way You Think:** Our posture plays a key role in our muscle and joint health. Our bodies have a certain alignment where they work best. When our posture is off, it leads to pain, disability, and loss of function.

In the next chapter, we'll look in more detail at the importance of the pelvis ...

Suggested Resources

Posture Alignment: The Missing Link in Health and Fitness, Paul D'Arezzo, MD, Marcellina Mountain Press, 2003. My earlier book provides a more in-depth look at posture and includes a detailed self-assessment and menus of exercises to help correct specific posture problems. www.posturealignment.com

CHAPTER **5**

The Pelvis

The pelvis, so called from its resemblance to a basin, is a bony ring, interposed between movable vertebrae of the vertebral column which it supports, and the lower limbs upon which it rests; it is stronger and more massively constructed than the wall of the cranial or thoracic cavities, and is composed of four bones: the two hip bones laterally and in front and the sacrum and coccyx behind.

—Gray's Anatomy

The pelvis is the largest bone in the body. It is the base on which the body's architecture is constructed. The pelvic bone supports and protects our internal organs and provides the platform from which we walk, jump, climb, and crawl. Like a central switching station, all the big muscles from above and below unite at the pelvis. Hence, the strength, flexibility, and alignment of the muscles surrounding our pelvis are crucial for optimal functioning of the body as a whole.

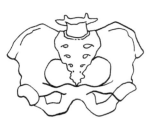

We Don't Want To Be Spilling Forward Or Backward

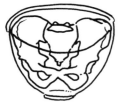

Pelvis means "basin," and the pelvic bone itself has a concave shape almost like a bowl. Ideally, we want the basin or bowl that is our pelvis to be anatomically level and things not to be spilling out in either direction.

Stand up and place your hands on your pelvic brim, fingers pointing straight ahead, thumbs pointing toward the rear. Now, without moving the rest of your body, tilt your pelvis forward so that your fingers move more toward the floor, and your pelvis tilts forward, and there is more of a pronounced arch in your low back. Your stomach should bulge forward. This is a forward-tilted pelvis.

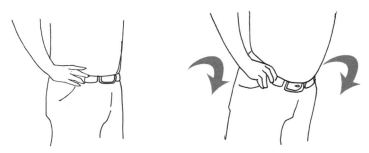

A person with a pelvis that is tilted or rolled too far forward will tend to have an exaggerated curve in their low back. That is, there will be too much arch in their low back. A forward-tilted pelvis also exaggerates the paunch in our midsection; our belly tends to spill over our beltline. One clue for a forward-tilted pelvis is to look at your belt. When standing upright, if your belt is tilted forward and down rather than being close to level, your pelvis is probably tilted forward.

A person with a forward-tilted pelvis may also look and feel as if they are falling forward—which indeed they are. Our bodies often compensate. We arch our low back even more and bring our shoulders back like ballast to counteract our fall forward.

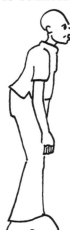

A forward-tilted pelvis can alter our gait, the way we walk. Our legs, instead of being aligned in a forward direction, are often rotated outward with our feet flared out to the side almost like a duck. We may walk with more of a waddle swinging one and then the other leg out to the side before bringing them forward.

Many people with a forward-tilted pelvis become virtually locked in this position. They lose much of the ability of their pelvis to tilt backward, and as years go by, the pelvic tilt forward becomes even more pronounced. Some arch in our low back is normal and desirable. With a forward-tilted pelvis, the arch may become overly pronounced leading to back and hip problems.

A backward-tilted pelvis presents the opposite problem. It is often a little more subtle and harder to recognize at first.

Stand up and place your hands on your pelvic brim again. This time tilt your whole pelvis backward jutting it slightly forward and flattening the curve in your low back. A person with a backward-tilted pelvis often appears as if they are sitting and collapsing downward in their low back even when they are standing.

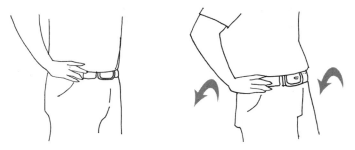

Whereas a forward-tilted pelvis is often due to excessive tightness of muscles (primarily the psoas muscle), which connect our thighs to our pelvis, a backward-tilted pelvis is often due to relative weakness of our pelvic musculature.

A lifestyle where we sit a lot contributes to a backward-tilted pelvis. In particular, every time you slouch down in a chair allowing your low back to push backward, you reinforce a backward-tilted pelvis.

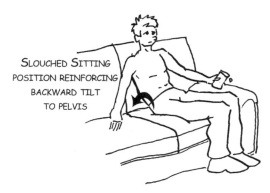

SLOUCHED SITTING POSITION REINFORCING BACKWARD TILT TO PELVIS

With a backward-tilted pelvis, the shoulders often roll forward, again in compensation—this time to keep from falling backward.

> For optimal function, our pelvis should be close to level. Like Goldilocks and the Three Bears, too much or too little tilt can lead to problems.

Cushy Couches And Chairs

If you've been to a furniture store lately, you may have noticed it's hard to find a couch that supports your body in an upright position. There are more and more cushy monstrosities that we collapse into or rather are absorbed into. Many chairs are similar. They encourage and foster a slumped position.

While this furniture is comfortable, it forces us into a backward-tilted pelvic position, and reinforces and strengthens the muscles that make that persist.

Many of us simply don't have the strength in our low backs and abdomens to sit upright any longer, and a vicious cycle is created. We demand and find comfortable furniture that allows us to stay in our backward-titled pelvic condition, and the weakness worsens.

Side-To-Side Tilt

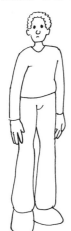

One side of the pelvis may also be higher or more forward than the other. Stand in front of a floor-length mirror and look closely at your hips. Is one hip slightly higher than the other? Since pull or stretch in one area has to be transmitted to other areas (remember the Tensegrity section in Chapter 2), look at your shoulders. Along with a tilted pelvis, one shoulder, either on the same or opposite side, is often slightly higher or lower than the other.

If you looked at someone with a tilted pelvis from the side, one hip often appears more forward than the other. In a sense, with a tilted pelvis our body is being rotated slightly around a central axis.

By definition, a tilted pelvis implies disparities in muscle strength and muscle flexibility from one side to the other. One side being tighter than the other produces the twist or tilt. Often, one side does more of the work carrying more of our weight than the other. There is often an imbalance in gait.

What causes side-to-side tilt? Any asymmetrical

muscle use-habit. Even such things as always carrying a purse over one shoulder or always standing with our weight on one hip may contribute to it.

Remember, we don't want ourselves in a situation where our weight isn't carried equally on both sides. This only tends to worsen.

> Our hips should be level. One hip or shoulder shouldn't be more forward, backward, higher, or lower than its partner on the opposite side.

Our Pelvis Has Got To Move

Even though we may not plan to dance like Elvis, our pelvises still need to move.

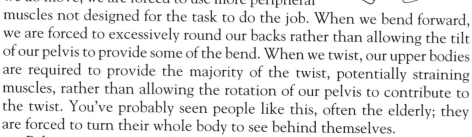

Along with being properly aligned, our pelvis also needs to be able to freely tilt forward and backward, side to side, and up and down. It is this freedom of movement at the pelvis that allows us to reach and bend, twist and turn, and walk. A perfectly aligned pelvis as described in the previous section means nothing if it can't also move.

A pelvis that can't move is like a stationary block of wood in the middle of our body. When we do move, we are forced to use more peripheral muscles not designed for the task to do the job. When we bend forward, we are forced to excessively round our backs rather than allowing the tilt of our pelvis to provide some of the bend. When we twist, our upper bodies are required to provide the majority of the twist, potentially straining muscles, rather than allowing the rotation of our pelvis to contribute to the twist. You've probably seen people like this, often the elderly; they are forced to turn their whole body to see behind themselves.

Pelvic movement is also necessary for proper walking. If you watch a person walk from the side, ideally their pelvis circumscribes an arch forward and backward and up and down. If you have problems walking, or with your feet, ankles, knees, or hips, correcting the alignment of your pelvis and restoring its movement ability can help.

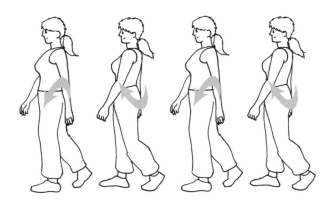

> Our pelvis has to be able to move. Along with the positioning of our pelvis, the ability of the pelvis to move freely is paramount to our overall muscle and joint health and function.

You've Got To Change The Position Of The Pelvis First

In the world of functional anatomy, the positioning of our pelvis more than anything else determines our posture. Alter even slightly the orientation of a person's pelvis—tilt it forward, backward, up, or down—and posture-wise, they become a different person. Because so many large and important muscles have their origins at the pelvis, weakness and tightness of these muscles in particular creates a cascade of effects that are distributed throughout the entire body.

> In the world of functional anatomy, the positioning of the pelvis in great part determines our posture and hence our function.

The alignment of our pelvis also in great part determines the curves in our back and hence contributes to a healthy back. How this relates to back pain is discussed in more detail in Chapter 12.

Small alterations in the alignment of the pelvis cause more dramatic alterations in posture as they are distributed up and down the linkages of our bodies. For example, if we change the carrying angle of the pelvis one degree, it can lead to a ten-degree alteration in the positioning of the shoulders or feet.

That's why exercises that work on the strength, flexibility, and alignment of our pelvic muscles are so important in correcting our posture. And attempts to correct our posture without addressing our pelvic and core muscles rarely lead to results.

For example, our shoulders may be hunched forward. Until and unless we first correct our forward- or backward-tilted pelvis, attempts to correct our shoulder positioning may be in vain.

Our pelvic muscles are also both big in the sense that they have the ability to override or usurp power from other muscles and in their potential to become *very tight*. If we only sit and walk, and rarely allow our pelvises any other movement, the muscles surrounding them become tight.

Pelvic muscles become very set in their ways. They don't yield easily to a changing of the status quo; they often don't readily relinquish their hold on our alignment. It takes concerted effort on our part to correct our pelvic positioning and alter our trajectory in postural alignment space. It takes time.

In the exercises that follow, be aware of this. Sometimes you need to do the exercises for several weeks for things to start to change on a permanent basis. By doing them regularly, you will feel a difference. Any small repositioning or change is a positive sign. Sometimes this occurs as a slight letting-go feeling deep in a joint, or an alteration in where your weight is being carried. That means things are working. Don't get discouraged.

> Pelvic muscles are big, strong, and often very tight.
> Pelvic muscles don't yield easily to change. It takes
> time.

The exercises that follow are a start to correcting the positioning of your pelvis. You are welcome to do any and all of them, but if you are noticeably tilted in one way or the other, you would benefit most by doing the prescribed menu. Also, do the exercises in the order prescribed; they build on each other.

Pelvic Exercises

<u>Forward-Tilted Pelvis</u>

What It Means: Muscles in front of groins too tight
Tight quads and hamstrings
Tight low back muscles
Often weak abdominal muscles

1. Astronaut
Page 163

7. Hamstring Stretch
with Strap
Page 173

2. Stair Drop
Page 183

8. Leg to Chest
Page 176

3. Cats and Dogs
Page 165

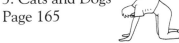

9. Lunge
Page 177

4. Downward Dog
Page 169

10. Abdominal
Crunches
Page 162

5. Japanese
Sitting Pose
Page 175

11. Imaginary Chair
Page 174

6. Child's Pose
Page 166

12. Groin Stretch
Page 173

Backward-Tilted Pelvis

What It Means: Muscles in front of thighs weak
Muscles surrounding pelvis weak
Hamstrings often too tight
Low back muscles often weak

1. Arm Circles
Page 163

7. Bridge
Page 165

2. Table Stretch
Page 185

8. Face Plant
Page 170

3. Cats and Dogs
Page 165

9. Pillow Squeezes
on Chair
Page 180

4. Hamstring Stretch
with Strap
Page 173

10. Squats
Page 182

5. Leg Lifts
Page 176

11. Groin Stretch
Page 173

6. Thigh Lifts
Page 185

Side-To-Side Tilt

What It Means: Disparity of muscle strength and flexibility side-to-side and back-to-front

1. Cats and Dogs
Page 165

6. Triangle
Page 187

2. Table Stretch
Page 185

7. Stair Drop
Page 183

3. Hamstring Stretch
with Strap
Page 173

8. Chair Twist
Page 166

4. Floor Twist
Page 172

9. Standing Bent-Knee
Chair Twist
Page 183

5. Face the Wall
Page 171
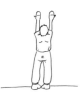

10. Japanese
Sitting Pose
Page 175

Exercises To Improve Range Of Motion Of The Pelvis

1. Cats and Dogs
Page 165

4. Child's Pose
Page 166

2. Table Stretch
Page 185

5. Downward Dog
Page 169

3. Couch Stretch
Page 168

6. Back Stretch
Page 164

The Way We Drive

Too fast. Too much. No, what I'm talking about is the fact that most of us spend a lot of time in our cars, and the way we sit while driving has the potential to either reinforce or be detrimental to correct postural alignment. When we drive, our bodies are placed in a habitual position, (for us) and we reinforce and strengthen this positioning by small muscular exertions. If it is a mal-aligned position, we reinforce and strengthen the muscles that would keep us mal-aligned when we leave the car.

When we drive, we use one foot (our right) more than the other. Often our right foot is splayed out to the side. When you drive, is one hip rolled forward of the other? Do you tend to always drive with one hand on the wheel with one shoulder rolled forward? How about your car seat? Are you slouched or slumped down in it (reinforcing a tilted-back pelvis) or more upright?

Become aware of your driving position. Make sure you aren't reinforcing faulty alignment with every mile you go.

Change The Way You Think: Pelvic positioning and the ability of the pelvis to freely move both have a decidedly important effect on posture and functional fitness. It takes time to restore alignment and flexibility to our pelvis, but it is a key aspect in our overall musculoskeletal health.

Okay, enough about the pelvis. It's my feet and knees that hurt—in the next chapter, we'll see why ...

Suggested Resources

Muscles, Testing and Function, Florence Kendall, Williams and Wilkins, 1993. A classic textbook providing a good foundation on how muscular strength and flexibility affect posture and movement.

CHAPTER 6

With Every Step We Take

> *As the body moves forward, one limb serves*
> *as a mobile source of support while the other*
> *advances itself to a new support site. Then the*
> *limbs reverse their roles. For the transfer*
> *of body weight from one limb to the other, both*
> *feet are in contact with the ground. This series*
> *of events is repeated by each limb with reciprocal*
> *timing until the person's destination is reached.*
>
> —Perry, *Gait Analysis*

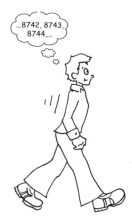

...8742, 8743, 8744,...

Yikes! Sounds pretty complicated. That said, the average person takes eight to ten thousand steps a day. That's a lot of steps.

And every step we take both reveals our body's alignment and reinforces it. Our gait reveals our individual gestalt of tight, weak, and strong muscles, and our own personal way of using them. Wherever our alignment is off, it will show. We can't hide it.

And every step we take reinforces and hammers this home step after step after step.

> Our gait—the way we walk—both reveals and
> reinforces our body's alignment.

Sit down on a park bench or in a mall and watch people walk by. Is their gait balanced? Does one side move the same as the other? Does their walk look smooth and graceful? Do the right foot and left foot strike the ground evenly with a steady cadence like the beating of a metronome— right, left, right, left?

Or, more likely, is there imbalance? Does one side swing forward slightly faster than the other? Is there excessive rocking? Does one side seem to do more of the work than the other (the other side coming along for the ride)? Do the arms swing evenly or does one arm swing more than the other? Is there a noticeable tilt to the pelvis, that is, one hip looks higher or more forward than the other? Is the cadence more like right, l-e-f-t, right, l-e-f-t?

Now walk down a long hallway (preferably wearing some loud clickety shoes) and feel and listen to your own walk. Is your own gait balanced? Irregularities in gait tell us that there are disparities in muscle strength, flexibility, and alignment from one side to the other. One side or one group of muscles is doing more work than the other side; or tightness and weakness of muscle groups is preventing us from using the muscles we're supposed to when we walk.

Not using the muscles I'm supposed to? Doesn't everyone have to use the same muscles? Not really. Many of those strange walks you witnessed while sitting on the park bench were the result of the body jerry-rigging solutions to get the job of moving done. We use different muscles to avoid putting pressure in certain areas. We use different muscles because the ones that should be doing the job are weak. We use certain muscles because other muscles have become too stiff to move the way they should.

> If your gait is off, it means there are disparities in muscle strength, flexibility, and alignment.

Preserving Our Ability To Walk

Walking is man's best medicine.

—Hippocrates

Everything is within walking distance if you have enough time.

—Stephen Wright

As we grow older, we want to preserve our ability to walk at all costs. If there is one thing that will accelerate our slide down the downward spiral, it is limitation in our ability to walk.

Any imbalance in our gait can make it uncomfortable and simply no fun to walk. A knee, hip, ankle, or foot that hurts can make us not want to walk. All this leads to eventually becoming unable to walk very far or unable to walk at all!

A good friend of mine has a neuroma, an inflammation of a nerve in the bottom of her foot. Because it is painful, she has stopped taking her daily walks. Unless something is done about the neuroma (perhaps surgery or orthotics), she will become even more inactive. Inactivity begets further inactivity. Soon muscles will weaken, and she will be *unable* to walk very far regardless of the neuroma. Soon her hip or back may start hurting. As I said in an earlier chapter, we want to prevent any break in our musculoskeletal armor. Any limitation in our walking ability is a big one. If a hip, knee, or foot is giving us problems for whatever reason, we need to do all we can to correct it. Don't let anything cause you to relinquish your ability to walk.

> Not wanting to or being unable to walk is a major risk factor for the downward spiral in our musculoskeletal health.

> Our ability to walk comfortably is something we want to maintain at all costs.

Problems with our gait also tend to worsen. Once we get a glitch in our gait, it tends to stay there or often to get worse. We may *learn* to walk in a way that avoids putting pressure on a tender area, but that causes problems elsewhere. A little favoring-of-one-side becomes a limp over time. A little limp or hobble becomes a big limp as the years go by. Pretty soon we opt for a cane to give us some support, or we avoid walking as much as possible. Sometimes there are things we could have done to correct these things before they caused serious problems.

> Little limps in our gait eventually become big limps.

Ideally, our gait should involve a cascade of muscles from our pelvis extending all the way down to our feet. Go back and observe a few more people on the street. They don't actually walk; they waddle. I don't say this to be derogatory but if you watch carefully, you will see they initiate the walking movements from their hips alternately swinging each thigh forward. Their lower legs, their calves, ankles, and feet don't do much of the work; they simply swing forward and clump down where they land. The hips and knees take a pounding with each step, and this is why people eventually say "Drop me off closer, that's too far to walk."

> By correcting our gait and our alignment, we have the opportunity to reinforce correct body mechanics with every step we take.

All the exercises in this book contribute to improving your gait. Along with that, here are a few other specific things you can do.

- Walk with your feet pointing straight ahead or close to it. Particularly when walking up or down stairs, try to keep your feet pointing straight ahead. Make sure both feet are pointing in the same direction, and that one is not flayed out to the side.

- When you walk up or down stairs, don't use your hands to assist you. Demand that your legs do the work. For most of us, one side is weaker than the other. Make sure your weak side does its fair share of lifting your weight.

- If you always carry a purse or backpack over one shoulder, carry it on your back or on the other side. Anything we do day after day tends to become ingrained in muscular psyche. Always carrying a bag on one side can contribute to a shoulder and hip tilt.

- Remember, if your knees, hip, feet, or ankles hurt, it may very well be caused by one of our three friends—muscle weakness, stiffness, and mal-alignment. Do all you can to correct these things.

- Become a walker. Take every opportunity to walk. And when you walk, focus on developing an even stride. Strive for an even cadence and allow your arms to swing freely.

Again, are all problems with our gait caused by stiffness, weakness, and mal-alignment? No. But these three things, if not the cause, certainly contribute to the demise of our walking ability. They are problems we can do something about, and thereby often prevent more extreme problems and solutions later.

Our Feet

> *Feet are tattletales.*
>
> —Ida Rolf

Our feet and our shoes in particular reveal disparities in gait and alignment. Where do your feet hurt? Where are there corns and calluses? Where are your shoes worn? Is one heel or the side of one heel more worn down than the other? Why?

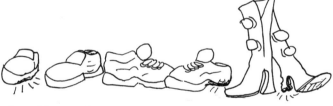

We tend to blame things on our feet. But what these things tell us is that our alignment, the alignment of everything above our feet, is concentrating the weight of our body more in those areas that are most sore or most worn. Our feet are simply on the bottom floor of the building and bear the brunt of any distortion in alignment from any of the upper floors. They compensate and adjust, they roll in and out, they tilt. They develop areas of increased pressure.

If we were tall skyscrapers, the weight of all the upper floors—instead of evenly being distributed throughout the entire base of the structure—would be concentrated on just one corner or edge of the building.

Is it any wonder one of our heels hurt, or we have pain along the edge of one foot? And that no number of foam pads ever really solves the problem. That's why thinking the problem is limited only to our feet, and using orthotics or having foot surgery may sometimes be ineffective long-term. Many of our foot maladies—bunions, corns, calluses, hammer toes—have their roots in uneven weight distribution. And if we don't break the cycle of improper weight distribution, the forces that created these problems will persist and, hence, so will our maladies.

Ideally, we want our weight to be equally distributed on both feet when we stand. And, for each individual foot, we want our weight to be evenly distributed front to back and from side to side.

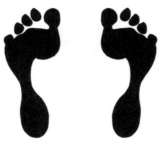

Where is the mal-alignment that causes our feet to hurt or our shoes to be unevenly worn? It can be anywhere from our feet to the tops of our heads or, more often, some combination of these areas.

For example, what would cause one foot to point out to the side and not the other? Think of a stack of blocks. To keep it simple, each block in sequence represents our pelvis, our thigh bone, our knee, our leg, our ankle, and our foot.

Pelvis

Thighs

Knees

Legs

Ankles
Feet

Rotation, a slight tilt in the carrying angle, at any of several locations could cause one foot to point outward.

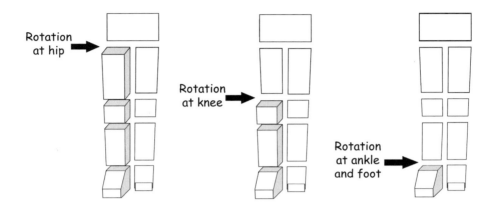

The mal-alignment may even be some combination of the above. But, wait, before you throw your hands up in frustration ("This is all too complicated!"), let me say this—it really doesn't matter. It doesn't matter *where* the problem is because with most of the exercises in this book we work on correcting everything.

Here are exercises that stretch, align, and strengthen the muscles in our lower extremities. Read the instructions in Chapter 13 carefully. When you can't stretch the same on one side as on the other, ask yourself why? The fact that you are tighter on one side than the other is a clue as to why your weight is not evenly distributed on both feet.

Overall Lower Extremity Exercises

Do these in order—

1. Cats and Dogs
Page 165

7. Side-Lying
Leg Lifts
Page 181

2. Stair Drop
Page 183

8. Pillow Squeezes
on Chair
Page 180

3. Hamstring Stretch
with Strap
Page 173

9. Toe Raises
Page 186

4. Crossover
Hip Stretch
Page 168

10. Standing Bent-Knee
Chair Twist
Page 183

5. Floor Twist
Page 172

11. Wall Bench
Page 188

6. Japanese
Sitting Pose
Page 175

12. Groin Stretch
Page 173

Orthopedic Braces

Not always, but sometimes, it is useful to rethink the use of these stabilizing devices. If there is true underlying ligamentous instability, a brace may provide necessary support to prevent further injury. And certainly braces and splints are useful after acute injuries to allow damaged tissues a chance to heal. But if you are using a brace on a chronic basis to support an area just because it hurts, you have to ask yourself what is the true cause of the pain. Could it be that your body alignment is off or that certain muscles are weak and need to be strengthened, stretched, and aligned?

Using a brace or support on a chronic basis is, in effect, saying, "I'm accepting this as it is. I'm willing to accept the fact that this will not get better, and by doing this I will probably be allowing certain muscles to get weaker and risk the compounding effects of that weakness throughout the rest of my body."

When immobilized, our muscles lose strength at an alarming rate. A muscle that isn't used because it is supported by a corset or brace will grow weak; it doesn't need to do its job. It's like some guy down in shipping being allowed just to sit around all day.

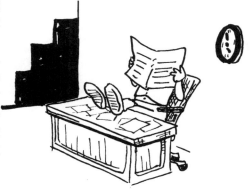

Pretty soon we may feel we can't get by without the brace and, indeed, we may have grown so weak that we can't. Is there something you can improve or correct so that you don't need the brace?

Weak In The Knees

If there is one place we particularly feel our mortality as we get older, it is in our knees. They creak, they strain, and they threaten to give out on us. Like questionable friends, we aren't sure they will be there for us when we need them.

Our knees are simply sentinels of the strength, flexibility, and alignment of our lower bodies. Our knees are where muscle weakness, tightness, and mal-alignment are felt. Our knees also take the brunt of the punishment from any abnormalities in our gait and from carrying around excess weight. Left unattended, all these things can contribute to arthritis or other knee problems

One of the recurrent themes of this book is that the location of a pain may not be its true source. Rather than focusing solely on our knees, a better question may be to ask ourselves what deficiencies in our strength, flexibility, or alignment could be causing or contributing to our knees hurting.

Pain or discomfort in the knees is very often due to weakness in our leg muscles. Because we walk and stand a lot, most of us assume our leg muscles must be strong, but many of us are much weaker in our leg muscles than we think.

> Our leg muscles are often much weaker than we think.

Our quadriceps muscles, those big bulky muscles in the front of our thighs, are primarily responsible for supporting our knees when we walk and step up or down. Our quadriceps act as a brake to support us and brace our knees when we walk so we don't *clump* down with each step, which is particularly damaging to the knee.

> Our thigh muscles are often weak and are unable to protect our knees.

Weak quadriceps muscles specifically have also been found to increase the risk of falls with age. In women weak quadriceps muscles are an independent risk factor for the development of osteoporosis.

Behind our thighs, our hamstrings brace our knees from the opposite side. These two muscle groups, quadriceps and hamstrings, are primarily responsible for supporting our knees when we walk.

So if your knees hurt, along with consulting your doctor when appropriate, also consider strengthening your leg muscles. And not just a little strong—make them really strong. For older people in a sedentary society this, more than anything, will result in a marked improvement in performing your favorite activities and in the quality of your everyday life.

> Strengthen those leg muscles.

There's one catch. All quadriceps and leg strengthening exercises are uncomfortable. They hurt and burn. Many exercise books give exercises that strengthen the quads. You try them once and go, "Yikes! No way! I ain't going to do that anymore!" So be forewarned. It has to feel uncomfortable and you have to hold the exercises long enough for them to feel uncomfortable. That means you're building strength.

> All leg strengthening exercises are uncomfortable.

If your knee, not your thigh, is terribly painful when you exercise, then stop. Adjust your positioning or try another similar, less-demanding exercise for now. See your doctor if the pain persists. Listen to your body, and use your best judgment. But consider that some discomfort, rather than being a sign to stop, may mean that you *really* need these exercises. Some of us have become so adverse to any strain on our bodies that we totally avoid any demand on our body, or think a little discomfort is dangerous or bad.

> Just because your knee creaks, feels like it's going to give out, or is wobbly or weak, isn't a reason not to do the exercises. It may mean that this is what you really need.

Dont's

There are several things you don't want to do with your knees.

You don't want to lock or hyperextend your knees. This can lead to overstretching the ligaments in your knee, leading to laxity in the knee joint and increasing your propensity for injury. The way to prevent this is to keep your quadriceps muscle *active*, keep a little tone and lift to your leg muscles, particularly when you are doing standing or balancing-on-one-foot exercises.

You also don't want to exercise in any way that creates torque or twisting force on your knee joint. If done improperly, many yoga postures can do this. The knee is a hinge joint in the frontal plane. In general, you always want your knee to be pointing in the same direction as your foot. You should adjust or modify any posture so that you don't feel the twist in your knee. Also, for the same reason, exercises such as the so-called hurdler's stretch, where your foot is flared to the side, puts excessive torque on the knee by stretching the ligaments and potentially damaging cartilage. A better variation is to always make sure your knees and feet are lined up and pointing directly behind you.

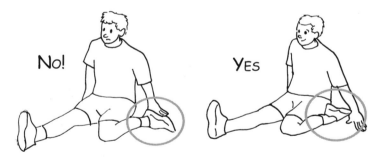

No!   YEs

Leg Strengthening Exercises

Any or all of these are good—

Warrior II
Page 188

Squats
Page 182

Thigh Lifts
Page 185

Wall Bench
Page 188

Imaginary Chair
Page 174

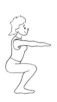

Reaching Down
Under
Page 180

Why Your Knees Hurt: Part Two

He's not fat, he's just short for his weight.

—Agnes Moorehead

You weigh too much. That puts inordinate amounts of strain and compression on your knee joints. Lose some weight.

Remember, increase in weight exponentially increases the forces placed on our knee joints. Lose some weight.

A New Habit

Make it a habit to stand up from sitting without using your hands to push off on the chair or on your legs. Point your feet straight ahead and stand using your leg and back muscles. If you aren't used to this, at first it might be difficult. You might have to weave and contort a little—all signs of weak leg muscles. Keep at it. This is a simple thing you can do every day that helps keep those muscles that support your knees strong.

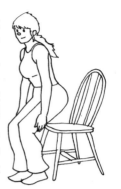

Change The Way You Think: Our gait both reveals and reinforces our alignment. Feet are tattletales. Weak leg muscles are responsible for much of our knee pain.

Now we're on a roll. The next chapter builds on this one. We look at the importance of staying strong ...

CHAPTER 7

Staying Strong

Getting strong now
Won't be long now
Getting strong now
Gonna fly now

—*Rocky,* "Gonna Fly Now"

There is no substitute for strength. There is no substitute to staying strong. Why do we want to stay strong? Because, to put it simply …

> It's our muscles that hold us up and allow us to do all the things we need and want to do.

Not bones, ligaments, tendons or skin. It's the strength of our muscles that holds up our skeleton and supports our posture in the gravitational slipstream that forever conspires to collapse us downward.

It's the strength of our muscles that supports our joints. Like shock absorbers, they absorb and attenuate impact on joints, preserving joint function and preventing and limiting the onset and progression of certain types of arthritis.

It's the strength of our muscles that allows us to do all the physical things we love and need to do now, and it is the strength of our muscles that will allow us to do all the things that we envision doing when we retire.

> Muscular strength is what protects our joints.
> Compromise in our muscular strength sets the stage
> for the downward spiral.

When our muscular strength begins to falter, like a gyroscope beginning to wobble, our entire musculoskeletal system is placed in peril. Loss of strength leads to pain, disability, and loss of function.

Where Is The Mystery?

Why do we lose muscular strength? Why do things that used to be easy to do become hard? For many of us, there is no mystery.

If we never get down on the floor and crawl under a table, is it any surprise that this becomes hard or impossible for some of us to do? Is it any surprise that we lose much of the strength and coordination to perform that movement?

If we never lift any significant weight with our arms or backs, is it surprising that the muscles needed to do that become weak? And is it really a surprise that we are prone to tear something or get injured on the rare occasion when we do lift something heavy?

If some of us sit for long periods of time—month after month, year after year—and never do anything to use the rest of our muscles, is it really surprising when our structure begins to collapse and we hurt?

Where is the mystery? If we very rarely use significant muscle strength to lift, pull, push, and carry very much, is it any surprise that our joints begin to hurt?

> How much of our loss of muscular strength and
> function is really simply due to lack of use?

Muscles are simpletons. If we use them, they remain strong. If we don't, they become weak. If we ask them to do things, they'll do it. If we don't, they just hang out.

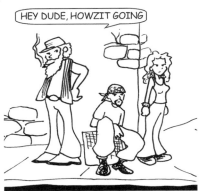

HEY DUDE, HOWZIT GOING

And how much of our chronic fatigue, generalized weakness, and just feeling tired is simply due to loss of muscular strength. It's an oxymoron but ...

> Some of our weakness may be due to …
> just getting weak.

One of the miracles of the human body is its ability to recover. With adequate stimulus, muscles are only too ready to jump back from even years of relative inactivity and regain their strength and tone. Given half a chance, our bodies, and our muscles in particular, are only too amenable to regaining their lost function.

> Strength, once lost, is not lost forever; but rather it is held in trust by our bodies until we are ready to rekindle it.

Loss Of Muscle Strength As Part Of The Downward Spiral

Loss of strength—

- Causes our posture to falter. Disparities in muscle strength—front to back and side to side—lead to alterations in compression and tension on other muscles and our joints. We don't look as young or feel as well as we should or could.

- Contributes to a loss of independence. We can't do as much physically as we used to. This need not be as dramatic as being in a wheelchair or using a walker. With loss of strength, we are more dependent on labor-saving devices to do things for us. We can't walk there. We can't do it ourselves. We hurt. When we lose muscle strength, our world grows smaller.

- Increases our risk of falls and fractures, both of which are leading causes of injury and disability in older individuals. By getting and staying strong, we increase bone density or at least limit the natural biological loss of bone density due to aging.

- Increases the wear and tear on our joints and puts us at increased risk for certain types of arthritis.

• Contributes to a decrease in our overall health. Our bodies are integrated wholes. The function and health of our hearts, lungs, spleen, and kidneys is directly related to our continual ability to move.

How Muscles Get Strong

> *Muscle is perhaps the most*
> *mutable of biological tissues.*
>
> —Carol Oatis, *Kinesiology*

Muscles stay strong by using them. Muscles get stronger by using them *more*. That's all there is to it. No big surprise.

> **To regain muscle strength, we have to do more than we are accustomed to.**

The catch for most of us who have lost strength is that we need to be *doing more*. We have to increase the demand on our muscles. And the most efficient, time-effective way to gain in muscle strength is to work a muscle close to its fatigue point, close to the point where it can do no more.

That means using the muscle close to the muscle's current limits of strength and creating that decidedly uncomfortable feeling of straining to hold ourselves up a few seconds longer or to do a few more repetitions of an exercise. If you do ten repetitions of an exercise, which repetition is the most important? The eleventh. It's that extra effort at the fatigue point where the gains in muscle strength are made.

> **It's the eleventh repetition that makes the difference.**

Lifting weights or doing repetitions of an exercise well beneath your limits—while beneficial—won't result in the increases in strength most of us need and are after. After all, you've come this far. Put in that little extra effort and maximize the gains for the time and effort spent.

> You have to fatigue a muscle for it to grow in strength.

Muscles gain in strength by several mechanisms. When an increased demand is placed on a muscle, it causes an increase both in size and in the number of muscle fibers (not necessarily resulting in an actual increase in bulk of the muscle). With increased demand, our muscles also become more efficient. On a cellular level, muscle metabolism improves. Neurologically, the muscles and the nerves controlling them also *learn* how to use themselves more effectively. The timing and firing sequences of muscle fibers are optimized, resulting in an increase in strength. That is why part of the gain in strength with strength training is independent of an increase in muscle size. This is also one of the reasons visualization is helpful for many high-level athletes. It helps program and reinforce the right firing sequence and coordination for the requisite physical activity.

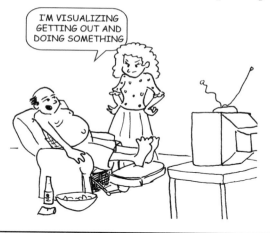

Resistance

To fatigue a muscle we need resistance, something for it to fight or hold out against. This can come in the form of holding your own weight up against gravity, repeating a desired movement over and over, pulling against an elastic band, or lifting actual weights. They all work.

Most of the exercises in this book use holding our own weight against gravity or repetitions of a simple movement for resistance.

Here are some key points to remember for any strengthening exercise.

First, remember the key rule of strengthening a muscle. You must place more demand on it than it is used to. You must work it to its limit.

You must fatigue the muscle. That means you have to either hold the exercise for long enough or do enough reps until it becomes hard to do it any longer. If you lift weight or do reps far below your limit, you won't gain much or any strength.

Be meticulous in your alignment. Don't compound your problems by slipping into bad habits that reinforce bad posture. At a local gym, one of the biggest mistakes I see people (guys in particular) making while lifting weights is not maintaining proper alignment. One foot is splayed to the side or their back is hunched over. Then they contort and twist their body to do a few more repetitions. If they aren't careful, they are simply creating stronger, more compact versions of their own dysfunctions.

> Don't compromise your alignment in order to impress people (or yourself).

Remember our rules of alignment for exercises. Unless stated otherwise—

- Make sure your feet are pointing straight ahead or close to it.
- Make sure your hips are level and not tilted. Be sure that one side isn't doing more of the work than the other.
- Make sure your shoulders are back and not hunched forward.

When you maintain correct alignment, you are reminding all the other muscles in your body, "This is the way I want you to hold yourself."

> Strengthening exercises are an opportunity to reinforce correct alignment. Take advantage of it.

> We want to reinforce correct alignment, particularly when we are in a loaded (weight-bearing) position.

When you are exercising and your alignment begins to falter, it's time to quit. Just for today. Even though you want to fatigue the muscle, you don't want to do it at the expense of contorting your posture or enlisting the help of other muscles you aren't trying to strengthen.

Let the muscles being addressed do the work. Often, certain muscles haven't been fully used in a long time. Certain exercises isolate them. We want the weak muscles to get the message that they are ones we want to come to life.

Remember, the reason we are forced to bob and weave and otherwise contort ourselves to get the job done is because the muscle we are trying to strengthen is already fatigued. Other already-strong muscles will want to help. We don't want the weak muscles to be up to their old ways of allowing other muscles to do the work for them. This may mean you can only do a given exercise for a few seconds or lift a small amount of weight. That's fine.

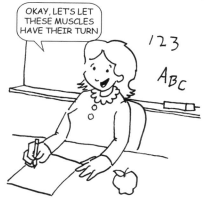

> Make sure you are working the muscle designed to be worked by the particular exercise you are doing. When you have to bob and weave, you've done enough.

> When your alignment begins to falter, you have done enough reps.

Make sure you go through the full range of motion with any exercise you do. Don't do truncated versions of the exercise where you only lift up halfway. Go to the extremes so that you strengthen the muscle throughout its full range of motion and preserve flexibility.

> Strengthen muscles throughout their full range of motion.

Do the strengthening exercises that you don't like. If you think about it, the reason you don't like them is because they demand that you use muscles that are probably weak. That's why it's uncomfortable or just plain hard to do those exercises. Those are exactly the exercises you should want to do and need to do.

> Do the exercises you don't like.

Weight Lifting

Along with the exercises in this book, many of us would also benefit from an actual weight-lifting program, using either machines or free weights.

> Many of us are much weaker than we think and would benefit from some industrial-strength strengthening.

Weight lifting often has negative connotations. Women fear they will bulk up and look like the women on the cover of body building magazines (don't worry—you won't). And men, after doing nothing for years, may be hesitant to even enter a gym.

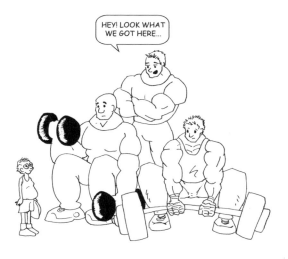

HEY! LOOK WHAT WE GOT HERE...

That said, doing the ten or twelve weight-machine circuit at your local health club two or three times a week can make a decided difference in your strength and overall musculoskeletal health. Light-weight dumbbells or weighted ankle and wrist belts are also good alternatives.

There are many good books that list simple weight-lifting exercises. Miriam Nelson's "Strong Women" series of books provides some of the best instruction, particularly for women. Or go to your local health club and get some instruction.

> Along with exercises such as the ones in this book, most of us would also benefit from a simple weight-lifting program.

> If you haven't lifted weights before, get some instruction and do it right.

Lots Of Little Muscles

There are lots of little muscles in our bodies. Some are small in size but play significant stabilizing roles for our spine and pelvis. Others are small in the sense that they don't share the fame of their more prominent brethren—biceps, lats, quadriceps—but nonetheless their strength and alignment contribute greatly to our overall musculoskeletal health. We need not know all their names. It's enough to know that there are a whole slew of smaller muscles that hold us upright, support our midsection and back, and allow us to transition gracefully from one movement to the next. These smaller muscles are particularly prone to atrophy with a sedentary lifestyle and aren't often addressed in many exercise programs.

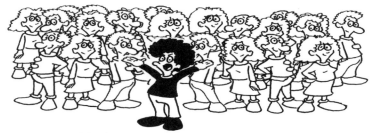

Hey! How about us little guys!

This is also why doing a half dozen weight-lifting type exercises, while beneficial, won't preserve the overall function we are after. Rather, we also need exercises and activities that seek out and address these hidden muscles. The exercises in this book are designed to address many of these little muscles.

Dead Spots

No, I'm not talking about those areas where you lose cell phone reception. Dead spots are locations in a movement sequence where we are weak, where little glitches in our strength force us to grunt a little or sweep past it because we can't support ourselves in that position.

For example, if you bend down to pick something up, you are probably fine as you start down and probably fine once you are all the way down. But there is a little spot in the middle where you don't quite have the strength to hold yourself up. That's a dead spot.

Dead spots are often due to weakness in core strength. Core strength refers to the deeper muscles surrounding our abdomen, pelvis, and low back. Pilates (pill-ah-teez), an exercise program focusing on core strength, describes these muscles as a corset around our middle. Ideally, all movement should be initiated from this central region.

In recent years many exercise programs such as yoga, Pilates, exercise ball classes, tai chi, and other core exercise programs, which recognize and address these core muscles, have grown in popularity. I heartily recommend any and all of them.

Here is a sampling of exercises that specifically address our core. Find a few of them that work for you and work your way up to doing the harder variations. You will notice a marked improvement in both your posture—you will hold yourself more upright—and in function. Such things as bending over and supporting yourself when you lean forward will become easier.

Core Strength Exercises

Add any or all of these to your exercise program—

Abdominal Crunches
Page 162

Side Crunches
Page 180

Bridge
Page 165

Lift-Ups
Page 176

Standing Airplane
Page 183

Clock
Page 167

Cobra
Page 167

Bow
Page 165

Locust
Page 177

Leg Lifts
Page 176

Boat
Page 164

Airplane
Page 162

Abs

If you go to a local gym, you realize we are obsessed with our abdominal muscles. There is no end to variations of abdominal exercises people do. There are even classes specifically devoted to just abdominal exercises. Everyone wants a flat midsection, and it seems every week on television there is a new ab machine.

While well-intentioned, it is useful to remember that what we are after is balance between muscle groups. And while we want strong abdominal muscles, we also want them to be resilient and flexible. We also want the muscles in our backs, which complement our ab muscles, to be equally strong. Are you putting in as much time with your back and side muscles as you are with your abdominal muscles?

Remember that some of the paunch in our midsections is from our collapsing postures. As you straighten up, some of that will go away.

Our abdominal muscles are made up of four distinct muscle groups. The exercises in the above core muscle section address these four groups. Here is a good way to stretch your abdominal muscles to complement the strengthening exercises.

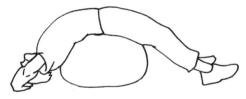

Balance

Balance is important in all aspects of our life—relationships, finances, work, and play. And exercises that demand balancing are equally important in our overall physical health and the health of our muscles and joints.

As we age, loss of balance puts us at risk for falls and injuries.

Balance involves a complex interplay of not only strength and flexibility but also vision, balance mechanisms in our ears and brain, and intact neurologic pathways throughout our body. Balance exercises help to keep all these systems intact, operational, and functional.

Trying To Balance Is What Improves Balance

It is our attempts at balancing that strengthens the muscles needed to …balance. It is the *trying* that improves our coordination. It is losing your balance, the constant little attempts to adjust and readjust while balancing, the wiggling of all those little muscles, that strengthens the muscles that are required for balancing.

> Attempting to balance is what improves and maintains all the systems required for balance.

No matter how good or bad you feel your balance is now, it doesn't matter. It is not about how well you can actually keep your balance at any given time. It is the attempts at balancing that matter. Over time, this is what will improve your balance.

Balancing exercises also require that both sides of the body do their fair share. For most of us, one side is better than the other. It may be easy to balance on our right foot, for example, our "good side," but much harder to balance on our left.

Remember, ideally the right side of your body should equal the left side when it comes to muscular strength and flexibility. Both sides need to be carrying their own weight. And the strength of the muscles in the back of our bodies should equal the strength of the muscles in the front of our bodies. Balance exercises are where we both test and, over time, correct this.

Balancing exercises also demand that we use those little core stabilizing muscles talked about earlier. Our attempts at balance strengthen and align them so that, if we are ever in a precarious situation, they are more likely to support us.

Balance Exercises

Add any or all of these to your exercise program—

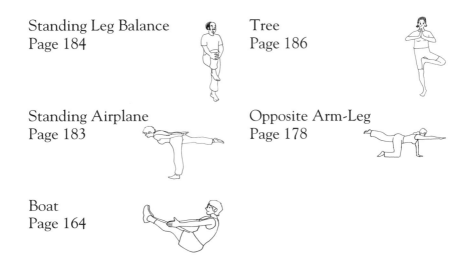

Standing Leg Balance
Page 184

Tree
Page 186

Standing Airplane
Page 183

Opposite Arm-Leg
Page 178

Boat
Page 164

If you don't have time to do the exercises (what!!!???), at least think of balancing as something useful to your overall fitness plan. Take every opportunity to balance, to stand on one foot when the opportunity presents itself, to reach and stretch for things, to walk on irregular surfaces that demand you to balance.

> Take advantage of every opportunity to balance.

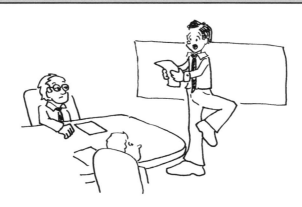

Change The Way You Think: Most of us are much weaker than we think. We need to get strong and stay strong. Muscular strength determines our alignment and protects our joints. Consider a simple weight-lifting program. Strengthen your core. Balance.

In the next chapter, we learn about the next link in our muscle and joint protection plan—staying flexible ...

CHAPTER 8

Staying Flexible

Race horses don't stretch,
so why should humans?

—Gordon Pirie
British middle distance record
holder of the 1950s

Good question? So why do I, an average man or woman, need to stretch or to be flexible?

We Live In A Box And It's Getting Smaller

The box I'm talking about is the area of personal space around us in which we can comfortably reach, stretch, bend, lean, and maneuver. It is our physical comfort zone.

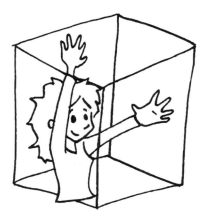

For most of us as we grow older, this box grows smaller. We can no longer stretch as far upward, reach as far backward, or turn as far to the sides. The arcs our joints circumscribe become more acute. Our world becomes smaller by degrees.

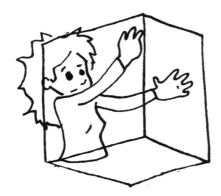
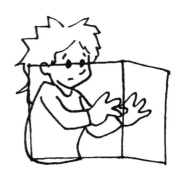

For some, the box has become so small that it now encompasses little more than a two-by-three foot area directly in front of us extending from our shoulders to our waist. Our steering wheels, phones, computers, and appliances all conveniently reside there. Anything outside this box becomes, if not a hardship, then certainly an inconvenience. "If it ain't in that area, then I ain't goin' to use it or get it." Or at least not until we move our whole body so that the object now resides in the box in front of us.

To explain it another way, let's say that the range of motion for one of your joints is sixty degrees. That is, your shoulder joint can circumscribe an arc of sixty degrees forward and back. With time, with lack of use, that arc becomes only fifty degrees, and then eventually forty degrees.

Now combine the effect of that one joint with all of the other joints. Imagine that they are undergoing similar curtailments in their ranges of motion. We become stiff and inflexible by degrees.

IF YOU CAN'T SEE MY MIRRORS. I CAN'T SEE YOU

Limitation in one joint's movement also contributes to other joints becoming less flexible. For example, if our hips are stiff and it becomes difficult to get down on the floor, then because of that we potentially lose much of the flexibility of other lower extremity joints. Our backs, knees, ankles, and feet become stiffer as a consequence.

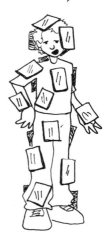

How far can you comfortably bend down toward your feet? How hard or easy is it for you to reach under a table where something has fallen and retrieve it? How easy is it for you to turn to the side to check your blind spot?

A great deal of this box-diminution is due to one simple fact.

> We are no longer required to reach or stretch very far; therefore, we don't reach or stretch very far. And because of that we lose much of the ability to do it.

Remember our maxim—use it or lose it. Our loss of flexibility didn't happen all at once. We started off as children with full ranges of motion able to reach up, down, back, and forth. But over the years as we reached and stretched, bent and leaned less and less, our ability to do those things diminished.

Now we are called upon to do some of these stretching activities on only the rarest of occasions—reaching up to put in a light bulb or to put luggage in an overhead compartment, twisting to reach far behind us, or crawling under a table to get something that may have fallen.

Our kingdoms have diminished in size. Restoring and maintaining flexibility is about restoring some of our sovereignty over these lost reaches of our kingdoms.

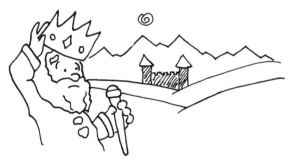

Things Get Tight And Stuck Together

With lack of use, body tissues truly become stuck together with a biochemical glue. This includes not only our muscles but all our connective tissue (skin, ligaments, tendons, fascia)—basically everything other than our bones.

It is the reason stroke victims' and spinal cord injury patients' joints must be routinely moved throughout their entire ranges of motion. Just as I said earlier, gravity conspires to leave us flattened, compressed, and close to the ground—well, not moving conspires to leave our joints, muscles, skin, and fascia glued together making us stiff and rigid.

Moving our joints through their full ranges of motion on a regular basis helps keep this glue from being created and from setting up. Movement keeps our joints lubricated and able to move. Some of the internal surfaces of our joints have no blood supply and it is the movement of our joints that allows nutritional support.

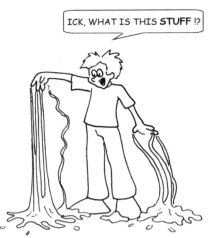

It's Tight Muscles That Hold Us In Our Awkward Positions

From Chapter 4, you already know it's tight, under-stretched, under-utilized muscles that hold us in our unique, individual postures. Until and unless we release our tight muscles, we will stay in our contracted posture. Rolled-forward shoulders and a hunched back will remain rolled-forward and hunched. Tight pelvic muscles will remain tight.

> Tight muscles are what hold us in our individual postures.

To gain the necessary space to reframe our posture in a more optimal way, we need to stretch these tight muscles. We need to regain the requisite amount of space to allow things to reposition themselves.

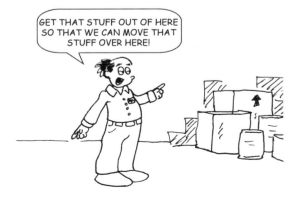

Flexibility Helps Prevent Injury

Each of our joints has an optimal range of motion—an area where it can optimally move and stretch. We want our joints to reside somewhere in the middle of their ranges of motion. Like a tennis player in the ready position, we want our joints to be able to go this way and that way and then return back to center.

> ## Tight muscles hold our joints in fixed positions.

A joint that is maxed out to one extreme or one that has no flexibility is an accident waiting to happen. It is like our tennis player being stuck on one side of the court or being unable to move to his left. There is no play in the joint, both literally and figuratively, setting us up for injury and making us unlikely to win at Wimbledon.

If one joint is locked in position and can't do its range of motion job, then the next joint up the line is called upon to provide movement. If that joint is also stiff, then the next joint further up the body is enlisted. Often they are requested to provide movement they aren't designed to provide.

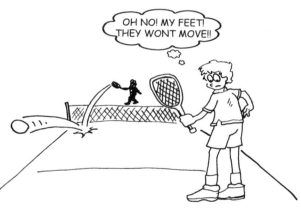

OH NO! MY FEET! THEY WONT MOVE!!

For example, if you've lost motion in your shoulder joint, the more vulnerable elbow and wrist joints will be called upon to provide movement best provided by the shoulder.

If tight muscles hold one of our joints locked to one side or the other, any demand on the joint out of the ordinary is more likely to cause something to pop, snap, rupture, tear, or fracture. A back that is frozen in one position is one that has lost its range of motion. If we are suddenly required to lift a heavy object or to bend forward, then something has to give. And it's usually not the groceries or the bag of concrete we are lifting.

Flexibility Helps Prevent Falls

With age comes an increased risk of falling. Falls cause fractures (broken bones) and other injuries. Hip fractures, in particular, are a major cause of disability and death in the elderly.

> You want to keep yourself flexible so that you're less likely to fall.

It is our flexibility that allows us to adjust and check our position and to catch ourselves before we fall. Compromised flexibility makes us into blocks of wood only too ready to topple over.

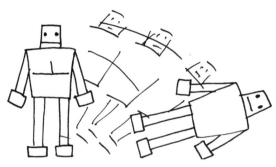

Flexibility And Strength Go Together

You don't want one without the other. It is the balance between strength and flexibility that holds us in correct alignment and allows us to do all the things we want to do.

Laxity of joints and hyper-flexibility *without* corresponding strength can increase our risk of joint injuries. Our muscles support our joints. Without enough muscular support, fragile ligaments not designed for the job are requisitioned to hold us up, making them prone to being adversely stretched or torn.

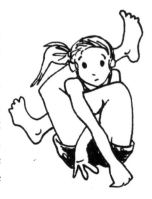

How Flexible Can We Become?

Each of our bodies has a level of flexibility drawn into its blueprint. Some of this is genetically determined; some of it is determined by what we did as children. Some people simply *are* stiffer than others. And within each individual body, there is variation. Some joints are stiffer and can never become quite as flexible as others.

But …and this is a big but. Before you blame your inflexibility on your grandparents ("You know, my grandmother wasn't very flexible either"), consider that most of us are nowhere near the innate levels of flexibility we are capable of. Most of us have lost vast amounts of our flexibility, which we are capable of restoring—if we want to.

Industrial-Strength Stretching

Stiffness sneaks up on us and many of us are very stiff. A half-hearted effort to touch our feet *way* down there ain't going to do it for us. A few stretches from a magazine article we read, while helpful, aren't going to give us back our lost kingdoms of movement.

> Many of us have gotten very stiff, and it's going to take industrial-strength stretching to restore our lost flexibility.

It takes a concerted effort to restore and maintain our flexibility. And muscles that have become stiff don't take kindly to efforts to change their routines and their limited range of motion. Our bodies have a physiological stretch reflex that kicks in to prevent us from stretching the muscles we are trying to stretch. Go figure. This safety mechanism actually tightens the muscle we are trying to stretch to prevent injury. It is the body's way of saying, "Do you really want to do this or is this an accident happening? Until I hear otherwise, I'm going to tighten things up to protect your joints and make sure no muscles tear."

To do our industrial-strength stretches, we have to override that reflex or at least sneak up on it enough so that it knows this isn't an accident and can relax the muscles we want to stretch. This is one reason bouncing stretching, along with being dangerous, isn't as effective as slow, controlled stretching such as in yoga.

Stiff Stuff

Two areas that commonly become tight as we grow older are our hamstrings (the muscles that run behind our thighs) and our calf muscles, which terminate in the Achilles tendon, the thick tendon behind our ankles. Tightness of the hamstrings in particular can severely limit movement as well as cause pain in buttocks and down the backs of our legs. Both the hamstrings and calf muscles are prone to injury if overly tight. Here are several exercises that stretch both these muscle groups. Try any or all of them—

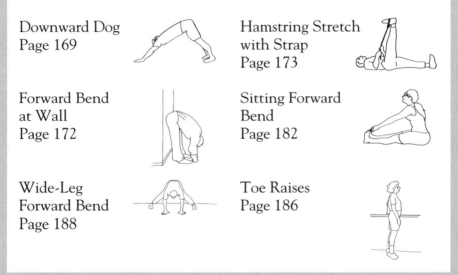

Downward Dog
Page 169

Hamstring Stretch
with Strap
Page 173

Forward Bend
at Wall
Page 172

Sitting Forward
Bend
Page 182

Wide-Leg
Forward Bend
Page 188

Toe Raises
Page 186

The Keys To Stretching And Regaining Flexibility

Five simple rules to remember—

1. *Warm up.* Don't just jump right in and start stretching to your limits. Do some gentle stretches first or go halfway for a few times and work your way into it. Combining the stretching exercises with the strengthening exercises in this book will also allow your muscles to get warm and more pliable. Stretching in a warmer environment is always safer than in a cool one. There is evidence that stretching with tissues at higher temperatures is not only safer but also leads to more permanent lengthening and less structural weakening.

2. Make sure you maximize getting the stretch where you really want it. You have to make sure you are doing a stretch in a way that really stretches the part you want to stretch. That is, you want to hold as many other areas of your body constant. You want to limit the amount of stretch absorbed by other joints and muscles, so that the stretch is focused on the area you want to stretch. That way, you get the most bang for your buck, the most results for your effort.

For example, if you want to stretch the quadriceps, the big muscle in front of the thigh, you don't want to lean forward so that the stretch is absorbed by the muscles in your pelvis.

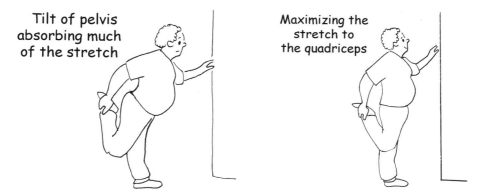

Tilt of pelvis absorbing much of the stretch

Maximizing the stretch to the quadriceps

Keep as many parts of your body constant so that you get the stretch where you want it. Don't let the wrong muscle groups absorb the stretch.

3. Stretch with correct alignment. Your body, my body, anybody's body will have a tendency to want to stretch in the directions of least resistance. Like fault lines in a rock, our bodies (our muscular psyches) will want to stretch in the direction they are used to stretching and which is easiest. But that won't help us, particularly if our posture is off. We want to make sure we are stretching in the direction of correct alignment. For example, it may be easy for us to bend forward if we allow our legs to roll out to the side. But correct alignment states that our legs should be aligned parallel, making the stretch more demanding and also fully stretching the muscles where we really need the stretch.

Don't compare how far you can go in a stretch with others or with some picture in a book. You will get far greater results by not going as far while maintaining correct alignment.

> To get the most out of your stretching, be meticulously aware of your alignment when you stretch.

4. *You have to really stretch.* Don't just go through the motions. You have to figure out for yourself where *your* limits are and carefully, gently but persistently, approach them and surpass them. This is an art and requires sensitivity on your part and listening to yourself. This is also one reason why it is probably better to do your stretches in a quiet environment so that you aren't distracted and can focus on and be conscious of what you are doing.

To make real progress, you have to stretch to the point where it is slightly uncomfortable—not painful—but where you really feel the stretch. And each day you stretch, you need to approach those limits again. Some days you will go farther than others. Some days you won't be as flexible as you were a few days before. Each day is different. Some yoga practices call this "playing the edges." This means mindfully approaching and hanging out in that uncomfortable area where you feel the stretch for you.

Can you hurt yourself—pull a muscle or injure a joint—by going too far? Sure. That's where you come in. Part of developing a stretching practice includes rekindling that sense of what is the point where you get results and what is too far for you.

How long to hold a stretch? Fifteen to thirty seconds is about right.

> Be careful but *really* stretch.

5. *Give it time.* Progress can be slow. Our flexibility varies each day and with the time of day. Sometimes it may feel we aren't making progress or are even going backward. Sometimes, even though we are doing our darndest to stretch one area, we feel we are making no progress. This could be because another area—another muscle somewhere else—is holding that area tight despite our best efforts. That's why the best stretching-flexibility approach is to do a series of exercises that stretch the whole body.

> Don't worry about the progress you are making.
> Worry about consistently stretching using correct
> principles.

Three Groups Of Stretching Exercises

In simplest terms, stretching exercises can be divided into three groups or directions: forward bends, backward bends, and twists. Add any or all of these to your execise program, or do them as groups on alternate days—

Bending Forward

Bending forward requires flexibility in three areas: our upper back, our pelvis, and our hamstrings.

Cats and Dogs
Page 165

Table Stretch
Page 185

Couch Stretch
Page 168

Child's Pose
Page 166

Hamstring Stretch
with Strap
Page 173

Forward Bend
at Wall
Page 172

Sitting Forward
Bend
Page 182

Wide-Leg
Forward Bend
Page 188

Bending Backwards

"I bend over backwards for you!" Well, after doing this series of exercises for a while you will be able to do that with more flexibility.

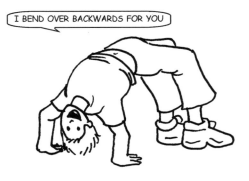

Back Stretch
Page 164

Bridge
Page 165

Cobra
Page 167

Bow
Page 165

Locust
Page 177

Airplane
Page 162

Twisting

We often forget about the sides of our bodies. We aren't machines with only a forward and a reverse. We live in a three-dimensional world.

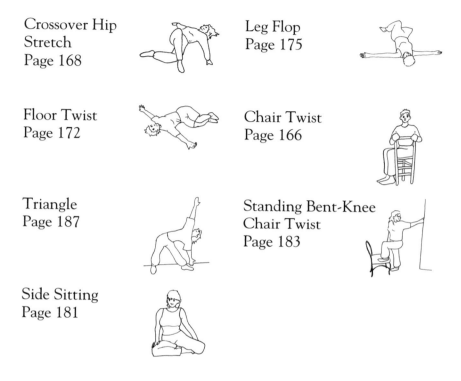

Crossover Hip
Stretch
Page 168

Leg Flop
Page 175

Floor Twist
Page 172

Chair Twist
Page 166

Triangle
Page 187

Standing Bent-Knee
Chair Twist
Page 183

Side Sitting
Page 181

Yoga

Yoga remains the premier stretching program commonly available in most communities. It helps to restore strength, alignment, flexibility, and balance. Most of the exercises in this book are taken from yoga. I heartily recommend yoga for everyone for a number of reasons.

- It is gentle.
- At its best, it is devoid of competition.
- It encourages us to listen to our own body.
- It requires us to use muscles we may not usually use and stretches us in directions we don't usually stretch. There are allegedly over 88,000 yoga poses.
- It helps to develop balance and core strength.

Here is a simple breakdown of a few of the types of yoga currently available.

Hatha Yoga—A generic term for all types of physical yoga.

Bikram Yoga—Also called hot yoga. This yoga is practiced in an overheated room. The same series of poses are repeated in each class. Be prepared to sweat. Some people like it; some find the heat to be too much.

Vinyasa Yoga—This type of yoga emphasizes flowing from one posture to the next coordinating movement with one's breath. It's fun and more dynamic than some of the more stationary types of yoga and gives more of a cardiovascular workout.

Iyengar Yoga—Could be called classic yoga. Places particular emphasis on the precision of the postures. Initially focuses on standing poses, which is beneficial for all of us.

Power Yoga—Involves a flow series of postures such as Sun Salutations along with more demanding strengthening and balance exercises.

> Excellent yoga instruction is now available almost everywhere. Take advantage of it.

Change The Way You Think: With loss of flexibility, our world becomes smaller. Flexibility protects our joints and helps protects us from falls. You have to *really* stretch. Take a yoga class.

In the next chapter, we look at the third part of our musculoskeletal protection plan—staying aligned ...

Suggested Resources

Science of Flexibility, Michael J. Alter, Human Kinetics, 2004 (3rd edition). An in-depth, scientific review of stretching and flexibility.

Although there are countless resources on yoga, here are two of my personal favorites.

"Yoga Journal's Yoga for Beginners with Patricia Walden" (video tape), Gaiam. An excellent starting tape; gets you off to a firm foundation.

Yoga, The Iyengar Way, Silva, Mira, and Shyam Mehta, Knopf, 1997. Beautiful pictures and detailed instructions.

CHAPTER 9

Staying Aligned

*The simple solution to all postural
and osteoarthritic conditions is to
avoid exercises in the direction towards
which the joint is bent and to exercise
in the opposite direction.*

—Victor Barker, *Posture Makes Perfect*

Correcting and maintaining our posture is perhaps the most unrecognized and underappreciated aspect of muscle and joint health.

> If our posture or body alignment is off, it becomes no longer fun or easy to do things; there is increased wear, tear, and strain on our muscles and joints; we don't look as young or healthy as we might; and we become more prone to pain, disability, and the downward spiral.

To be fair, most of us are not aware of what correct biomechanical alignment really is. We aren't taught it, and we aren't aware of the importance of it. We may have some vague sense that we should be more upright and less slouched but aside from that we often don't know exactly what is wrong. Or we may think that our posture is not that off or that little deviations in our posture can't make that much of a difference.

Most of us are more off than we think, and we don't have to be way off in our posture for it to have potentially catastrophic effects on our muscles and joints in the future.

Reread Chapter 3. Look at yourself closely in a mirror, both from the front and from the side. Or read my previous book, *Posture Alignment: The Missing Link in Health and Fitness* (Marcellina Mountain Press, 2003), which is devoted entirely to this subject.

The other reason correcting our posture isn't popular is that it's, if not hard, at least tricky to change our posture, and not many people know how to do it. Health and fitness books or magazine articles may make passing mention of correcting our posture saying such things as "make sure you stand erect," "pull your shoulders back," or "sit up straight," but even if we try to do these things, they don't produce any long-term change in our posture.

The other problem is that each day we are actually reinforcing our posture—whatever it is for us. If we are out of line, the muscles that are too tight have a tendency to become tighter. The muscles that are weak and aren't doing their job tend to stay weak. Strong muscles get more set in their ways and, in a sense, more confident of their supremacy. To change our posture we are, in a very real sense, fighting an uphill battle against the status quo.

> It takes a concerted effort to change our posture.

And if we just get out and exercise any old way, we risk reinforcing and perpetuating what we already have. Even if we become strong and flexible as in the previous chapters—we risk becoming stronger, more flexible versions of our crooked selves.

> If we simply exercise without addressing our posture, we risk becoming stronger versions of our crooked selves.

To change our posture we need to stretch the muscles that are tight, strengthen the muscles that are weak, and then put ourselves into correct alignment or as close to it as we can. This allows our bodies to begin to relearn to use a different, more appropriate set of muscles to hold ourselves up. Over time and by degrees, our posture improves.

A second key is to place ourselves in correct alignment in a *loaded* position. That means we want to support our weight or use our own strength to hold ourselves in that position. This *demands* that new muscles hold us there. It is the difference between correcting our posture while lying on a bed and correcting it while holding up several bags of concrete.

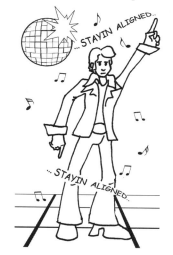

The exercises that follow are beneficial for everyone. There are several important things to remember.

The key to doing all of these exercises is to focus on doing them with correct alignment …I mean, that's why we are doing them. You are wasting your time if you just slop your way through them without purposely focusing on the positioning of your feet, hips, and back. If your posture is off, it *should* feel different or weird for you.

Correct alignment unless stated otherwise includes—

• Feet pointing straight ahead or close to it. Feet hip-width apart.

• Hips level. One hip shouldn't be more forward or lifted than the other. Be aware of this also in the supine (laying on your back) exercises; one hip shouldn't be cocked higher than the other.

• Shoulders back. A good way to remember this is to consciously lift your shoulders up, then back, and then drop them down.

• Low back in neutral. This means you want some curve in your low back; you don't want it completely flat nor do you want it excessively arched.

That said, it's obviously impossible to do the exercises with perfect alignment if your posture if off to begin with. Do them with the best alignment you can, constantly focusing on correcting and tweaking things to improve. There is also a tendency to slowly fall out of correct alignment as you hold a position or do repetitions. Be aware of this and correct your positioning when you begin to get off.

A few more tips—

• Get a small timer. That way you can accurately time how long you are holding each exercise and over time increase it. Without a timer, you end up guessing or looking at a clock.

• Read the instructions carefully. Some of the exercises may sound like exercises you have done before, but there are usually a few variations that make them more effective.

• Doing the exercises in the sequence listed is most effective. They build off of each other.

• It takes time to change your posture—weeks or months. But after doing the exercises even once, you should feel an alteration in your alignment. After doing the exercises, walk around. Notice if you feel your weight being carried slightly differently. Maybe you'll feel your weight more on one foot than it used to be, or feel as if you are using a muscle you aren't used to. All those things are good. That means things are working. Over time you will return to your old posture. But eventually these new changes will become home.

• Sometimes one part of the body can't change until and unless another part of the body changes. Remember how our body is linked together. For example, your shoulders may be rolled forward. Until and unless your hips begin to reposition themselves, you shoulders will be unable to fully return to their correct position. This occurs in starts and stops. One part gives up a little of its hold on the body, which allows another part to relax a little, which allows the first to relax still further. And on it goes. Most often this is felt as little micro-adjustments in your posture as you do the exercise, tight muscles relaxing and giving up a little of their hold.

Exercises To Improve Your Posture

Do this group of exercises in order. They build off each other.

1. Arm Circles
Page 163

7. Downward Dog
Page 169

2. Elbow Curls
Page 170

8. Hamstring Stretch
with Strap
Page 173

3. Overhead
Stretch
Page 179

9. Floor Twist
Page 172

4. Table Stretch
Page 185

10. Abdominal
Crunches
Page 162

5. Stair Drop
Page 183

11. Face the Wall
Page 171
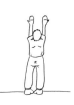

6. Cats and Dogs
Page 165

12. Floor Sit
Page171

continued on next page

13. Pillow Squeezes
on Chair
Page 180

15. Imaginary Chair
Page 174

14. Standing Bent-Knee
Chair Twist
Page 183

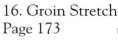

16. Groin Stretch
Page 173

Other Little Things You Can Do

Every day we also have the opportunity to reinforce correct alignment.
Along with the exercises, here are some simple things you can do—

- When standing in a grocery line or waiting for an elevator, make a
conscious effort for a few moments to stand upright with your feet
hip-width apart and your weight evenly balanced between both
feet. We often have our weight on either one side or the other
or are leaning against something. Just stand straight. You may not
get faster service, the elevator may not come quicker but you will
look and feel better and be doing something to reinforce correct
alignment.

- If you sit a lot, every hour or so make it a point to sit upright with
good posture for ten minutes—weight toward the back of the chair,
slight arch in your low back, shoulders back slightly, feet on floor
hip-width apart.

- When walking up or down stairs, walk with your feet pointing straight ahead. They don't have to point perfectly straight ahead (a few degrees out to the side is okay), but what we don't want is both feet splayed way out to the side or one foot out to the side and the other foot straight. This begins to help align the muscles in your legs and hips.

- Look at other people's posture. Look at the way they walk, stand, move, and sit. Look at how young or old they are, listen to their health complaints. Think about how much of this might have something to do with their body alignment. Learn more, read more, become more aware of the importance of our body's alignment.

> **Change The Way You Think:** Our posture or body alignment is the missing link in muscle and joint health. Along with getting strong and staying flexible, correct and maintain your body's alignment.

In the next chapter, we'll begin putting everything together—how and why we need to stay active ...

Suggested Resources

The Egoscue Method: Most of the posture exercises in this book and the logic behind them are taken from the books and work of Pete Egoscue. I heartily recommend all of his excellent books on body alignment. He also has clinics in San Diego and at several other locations throughout the country where individual therapy is available. Visit the website: www.egoscue.com

CHAPTER 10

Staying Active

*Generally speaking, all parts of the body which
have a function, if used in moderation, and
exercised in labors to which each is accustomed,
becomes thereby healthy and well-developed, and
age slowly; but if unused and left idle, they become
liable to disease, defective in growth, and age
quickly. This is especially the case with joints and
ligaments, if one does not use them.*

—Hippocrates

To put it simply—

> Those who are physically active tend to remain
> physically active.

Things work best when used. Cars, machinery, personal skills—it's the same with our muscles and joints. Use them as much as possible. Put them through their paces whenever you get the chance. Being physically active *now* is the fuel that will keep us physically active in the years to come and help prevent a host of muscle and joint problems.

When we lose or relinquish physical activity, our world becomes smaller. There are fewer things we can do or we can't do them as long. Our physical body becomes a limitation in deciding whether to not to go somewhere or do something.

> Staying active is a high-yield activity now and in the
> years to come.

Just as a diet of junk food leads to more health problems down the road, a diet of inactivity leads to more movement problems down the road. If you aren't moving much now, or your movement is limited to going from the bed, to the car, to the desk, to the table, to the car, and to the bed again—it is only going to get worse. That is the sobering fact that should spur us all into action. And I mean physical action.

Do It Yourself

We are upright, load-bearing, all-terrain, all-weather motion machines.

—Pete Egoscue

In a world that day by day demands less and less of us physically, we have to make a conscious effort to seek out and take advantage of opportunities to use our bodies. We have to swim against the tide of decreasing physical demand and keep doing things physically even when there are opportunities that may make it easier (less movement) for us.

> If you live a predominately sedentary life, then you have to take active steps to remain active.

Remember the man in one of the earlier chapters who was trying to figure out how to do the most with the least amount of physical effort. Well, if we want to preserve and maintain our muscles and joints as long as possible, then we have to be aware of that tendency and take steps to thwart it. As much as possible, do things yourself the physical way by using your own hands, shoulders, legs, and feet.

> Do things yourself the physical way when at all possible.

There is also a tendency for some people to think of physical activity as beneath them. After all, our parents or grandparents may have struggled at physical jobs their entire lives so that we could go to college and be free of that. We are now sophisticated enough and rich enough that we don't have to physically do much anymore. We can have people and things do stuff for us. Mechanical devices open doors for us and whisk us up to the mountain tops of buildings with no effort on our part. We hire other people to cut our lawns and do our physical work for us, rationalizing that we are too busy or important now or that physical labor is beneath us.

When we do this, we deny our biological heritage. We are like birds saying they no longer need to fly, or fish saying they no longer need to swim. Like bastard children, we want to cover up or deny our parentage. But in a word, we are and remain animals. And like all other animals, we need to stay active to stay fully functional. "Move it or lose it," might as well be our battle cry as we move into the later years of our life. And when I say "lose it," I no longer just mean our ability to move but in a very real sense our health, our happiness, and potentially our lives before their time.

We also have to see the value of the variety of quirky movements we have an opportunity to do on a daily basis.

If Movement Is Good, Then Varied Movement Is Better

If we get the opportunity to stretch, climb, or reach over or under something in a manner we don't usually do, we should take advantage of it. Moving in ways we don't usually move stretches areas of muscles that aren't usually stretched. It provides lubrication to joint tissues that don't usually get it. It helps to prevent that nasty glue from setting up that would stick our tissues together if given half a chance. It provides blood and lymphatic flow to areas that usually get short-changed. It demands us to use muscles or cascades of muscles that usually don't get much or any workout. It provides demand and stimulation to our neurological system and our brains. Recognize the value of moving in ways you don't usually move.

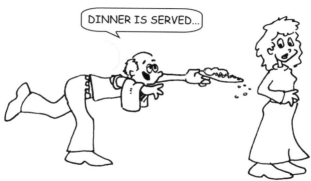

> If you don't usually move that way, then you should.

> Do things you don't usually do.

Recognize the value in lifting, stretching, reaching, and carrying. Recognize the importance of digging, crawling, getting down on the floor, climbing over and under things, twisting, turning, and putting our bodies in awkward, different positions. Don't be so quick not to carry something just because it's heavy. Don't be so quick not to do something because it is physically hard. All these things provide much-needed stimulation to parts of our body that otherwise may not get much use.

> Take every opportunity to reach, stretch, bend, lift,
> and carry things.

This means not giving up things such as raking or sweeping or cleaning things just because there is a new-fangled blower tool that can do it for you or you have the money to hire it out. This means painting, cooking, repairing it yourself, in part because of the motion it will give you. This means taking every opportunity to crawl under to get something, to climb over something, to lift, move, and carry things yourself.

This means walking as much as possible instead of driving. This means not giving up your favorite sport. This means trying new sports and activities because of the new and different demand they provide your body, regardless of how well you may initially perform at them.

For most of us, the fodder for improved physical being is there every day if we would but only reach out and take it. But we need to literally reach out and take it and carry it ourselves.

> Make it part of your mental persona to do things
> yourself (the physical way) as much as possible even
> if it sometimes takes more time or effort.

Think about your parents or grandparents. Most of us are aware of some older individual who remained active well into their later years. And more often than not, for whatever reason, they continued to do things themselves—to work in the garden, to walk up and down stairs, to carry laundry baskets, to clean their house themselves. It is all that movement that helped keep them alive.

Even the current trend toward ranchers or houses or apartments without stairs while convenient should give one pause. You don't want to give up going up and down stairs until and unless you absolutely have to.

Dylan Thomas, the Welsh poet, says to "Rage, rage against the dying of the light." Well, we have to rage, rage against the dying of the physical movement light. Don't relinquish movement in your life.

And to reiterate a theme that runs throughout this book—don't be so quick to blame difficulty in doing something on aging or some perceived flaw in your body.

> If you can't do something or it is hard, *first* consider that it may be because you haven't been doing very much for a while.

Victim Mentality

The media and a legal system that bombard us with people being supposedly wronged by the government, big business, or anyone else with deep pockets contribute to a victim mentality. It's not my fault. They did it to me. I didn't have anything to do with it.

This mindset can be fatal with regard to our health. There are things only *we* have both the ability and responsibility to maintain, and unfortunately once they get too far awry all the king's horses and all the king's men aren't going to be able to put us back together again.

As an aside, many so-called alternative medical therapies, while helpful, are palliative at best. Unless and until we address the underlying culprits—weakness, stiffness, and posture—we often risk more of the same.

> Take an active role in maintaining your muscle and joint health.

I doubt that you'd be reading this book if you felt this way, but some people think of it as almost a badge of honor to be disabled. Believe it or not, some people indulge in the aches and pains they associate with aging and corresponding disability. You don't want to be one of those people. I assume you already know this but remember—

- You don't want to get one of those little handicapped stickers or license plates and park up close unless you absolutely have to.

- You don't want to have any braces or supports on your body unless you absolutely need to. You want your own muscles to hold you up.

- You don't want to use a cane or a walker before your time.

- You don't want to drive around in a little electric-powered cart at Wal-Mart or the grocery store unless you absolutely have no other alternative.

> Disability begets further disability.

Less movement begets further loss of movement. Things get stiffer, tighter, weaker, and more out of line. If you can't do it now, you will be able to do even less as time goes on—if you aren't vigilant.

The Perfect Office Chair

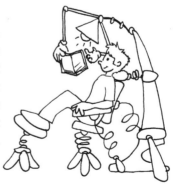

The type of office chair you have and the level of your computer *can* make a difference in your comfort level at work—up to a point. But don't get overly caught up in more and more ergonomic solutions to problems at the expense of avoiding what is often the real cause—weakness, stiffness, and mal-alignment.

Sports

And whatever sport or activity you participate in, let me tell you right now—

> ### It's too early to give up doing that.

Whatever it is. Walking, hiking, playing tennis, golf, squash, biking, dancing. Whatever it is. It's not time yet. I'll let you know when. I'm being a little tongue in cheek here, but what I mean is—once we give up or stop doing activities, we risk giving them up forever. Remember, you may live much longer than you think. And you may look back and think, "Jeez, I wish I would have kept doing that."

And if you don't participate in any sport, no matter what your age, consider taking something up. No matter what your skill level, there is great value in chasing a tennis ball around a tennis court. It's not about how good you are. It's about the physical movement the activity entails.

> ### It's the running around and moving we are after.

Even better, find a friend or partner who also understands the importance of varied activity. Hike. Bike. Dance. Go to a driving range and hit golf balls. Play ping pong. Go bowling.

Because we are constantly exposed to such high-caliber athletes on TV, many of us are self-conscious and prone to not even participate. If we aren't careful, this can be our undoing.

I mean, you know, after all if I can't be a world-class athlete, why bother!

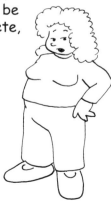

Or we may think that if we can't do it as well as we used to, then what's the point. Or we may simply feel that we just aren't athletic. We never were athletes and don't expect to be. But it's not about that. It's about taking advantage of opportunities to move.

Move.

The Importance Of Stairs

Elevators, escalators, moving walkways, ranch houses—many of us live in an environment that is becoming more and more devoid of stairs. And if we aren't careful, we can go days, weeks, and months without having to climb up or down any significant incline. Is it any wonder that our quadriceps and hamstrings grow weak, our posture deteriorates, and we become prone to hip and knee problems?

Stepping up and stepping down provide necessary demand and loading for our weight-carrying joints. Finding and using stairs and walking up and down hills, are easy solutions that give added stimulation to oft neglected muscle groups.

Take advantage of walking up and down stairs every chance you get.

Walking up and down stairs is also a chance to improve your alignment. Walk *both* up and down stairs with *both* your feet facing straight ahead. Usually one or the other flares out to the side, reinforcing a tilt or twist to our body. With your feet straight, you'll immediately notice yourself having to use different (more optimal) muscles. And let your legs do the work. Don't push off on your legs or use a railing.

Here are two exercises that both test and allow you to strengthen your stepping-up-and-stepping-down muscles.

Step-Ups and Step-Downs

Find a box, bench, chair, or low table that you can step up on. Something about eighteen inches high is perfect. Step up onto the bench using your right leg until you are standing on top of the bench with both feet. Don't push on your leg with your hands or bounce to get momentum. Let your leg muscles do the work. How hard or easy is that to do?

Next, turn around and step down again leading with your right foot. Don't jump but step down. Can the muscles surrounding your knee and hip adequately stabilize you?

Now repeat on the opposite side. Work your way up to doing twenty on each side each day.

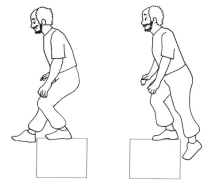

Make it a point to walk somewhere that has a few hills, every day, or walk up and down stairs.

An Exercise Program For You

People who live sedentary lives
urgently need exercise.

—Hieronymus Mercurialis,
16th century

Hieronymus Mercurialis was right. To put it another way, if you live a predominantly sedentary life, after a certain age you are either actively taking steps to maintain your muscles and joints or you are not. If you are not, you will probably fall prey to the downward spiral at an earlier age. That's all there is to it.

For most of us, this means finding or designing an exercise program we do on a regular basis—something that works for us. The exercises in this book are a good foundation.

Here are some more tips—

- It's better to do less and do it regularly than to go all-out for a short period of time and then quit. Think of your exercise program as something you will do now and, with modifications, for the rest of your life. If you can only do a few minutes every other day, that's fine. As you regain and restore function, you may want to do more.

- Vary your activity. Try to avoid doing only one sport or activity over and over and over. For example, if you walk or run, try to make time for some exercises that address your upper body.

- Sometimes the fact that we don't have the time to do a full activity keeps us from doing anything. Instead, try to intersperse your day with little segments of physical activity. Consider taking a brisk walk around the block during lunch, play tennis for only twenty minutes or throw a Frisbee around in the backyard for a few minutes. All these things add up.

- Although this book isn't about cardiovascular fitness, do something where you get at least a little out of breath. If you think about it, just as with our muscles and joints, if we never use our hearts or lungs anywhere near their limits, is it surprising when they lose some of their resiliency and functional reserve. It's a good thing to pant a little.

- Break up your routine. One day do stretching exercises, the next day lift weights, the next day go for a long walk. Don't get stuck in a routine where you do the same thing over and over and over.

- Give preference to exercises where you use your whole body rather than just one area. Give some preference to exercises with linked movements.

- Consider doing the exercises that you don't like. By definition, your body is telling you that you are weak or deficient in the strength, flexibility, or alignment required to do those exercises. They are often the ones you need to do.

- Listen to yourself. Listen to your own body. We are all much smarter than we think we are—if we listen to ourselves. Most of us know what we need and how to go about doing it.

- Not always but sometimes when you hurt it means you physically need to do more, not less. Sometimes our muscle and joint hurting is a sign of not doing enough and of things growing weak or stiff and putting pressure where it shouldn't be. Listen to your body; treat it kindly. Be gentle; don't force things. When we exercise, all that hurts or feels uncomfortable or requires some strain or effort isn't bad. Sometimes we're a little too quick to say it hurts and stop. Sometimes a slight uncomfortable feeling is part of the pathway to no pain.

> Consider the possibility that some of your muscle and joint pain may be a signal of the need to do more physically, rather than less.

- Make sure you do exercises on both sides of your bodies. We live in a right-hand dominant world. But our left side isn't just along for the ride. Remember, it is the balance of muscular strength, left-to-right, back-to-front, that contributes to proper posture. Make sure your non-dominant side has an opportunity to do its fair share of the work.

- Do balance exercises (Chapter 7) or activities that demand balance.

- Allow your body to figure things out. If you can't immediately do a physical activity, sport, or exercise, don't immediately criticize yourself or feel like you are lacking in something. Your attempts at trying to do it are what allow your body to figure out the correct muscular sequence for you. Let your body try it out in different ways. Think of children doing cartwheels on a front lawn. They fall over this way and that. They experiment, they laugh. They let their bodies figure things out.

- What you may have done in the past exercise-wise may not be what you need now. Many of us have a favorite sport or activity we used to do in college or when we were younger. We think that to get back in shape we need to do that again. So we get out the jogging shoes and try to run again, or start lifting weights like we did when we were in our twenties. Consider the possibility that what would help you the most may not be what you did in the past. Most people would benefit more from exercises similar to the ones in this book.

- Beware of exercise fads and new machines. There is no substitute for strength, flexibility, and alignment. And one contrivance can't do all these things for you.

- Give high priority to posture, alignment, and correct body mechanics in anything you do.

Warning: Effort Required

If you haven't done much for several years, it's going to take some real effort to get back into shape. Age, increased weight, loss of strength, flexibility, and cardiopulmonary reserves all conspire to make it feel terrible when you make that first attempt to turn things around.

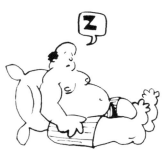

A body at rest tends to stay at rest.

Muscles have gotten set in their ways; certain muscles haven't been fully used in a long time. As you and I get older, it becomes harder and takes more effort—expect this. Gains are often less dramatic. Sometimes it seems that, even with a lot of effort, we are just holding our own. Expect that it's going to take some effort to turn things around.

Small Change

Small changes in the way we think *do* make a difference long-term. Changing your thinking to see the value of movement now will make a difference in who you are five and ten years from now. A little change now—a slight tweaking of our viewpoint—can make a big difference in function and preventing disability as the years of our lives play out.

A small change in our activity level *now*, when multiplied and compounded month after month, year after year, will make us into a different person physically than we would have been otherwise.

> Small changes in our activity level and the way we think about activity can make a difference in our lives long-term.

Change The Way You Think: Make it part of your mental belief system to do things for yourself the physical way. If movement is good, varied movement is better. Take advantage of sports and other organized physical activities. Develop an exercise program that works for you.

In the next chapter, we'll take a quick look at arthritis ...

CHAPTER 11

Arthritis

I don't deserve this award, but then I have arthritis and I don't deserve that, either.

—Jack Benny

Arthritis is the leading cause of disability in older individuals. One in seven or nearly 40 million Americans have some form of arthritis, and by 2020 it is estimated that 60 million people in the United States will suffer from it. Our parents may have been incapacitated by it. We may have it ourselves or worry that we may be developing it.

Causes of arthritis are complex but muscle weakness, inflexibility, and joint mal-alignment all contribute to the disability. While there are over one hundred different disorders encompassed by the word arthritis, the two most common types are rheumatoid arthritis and osteoarthritis.

Rheumatoid arthritis is an auto-immune disease, which means the body's own immune system goes awry and begins attacking its own joint tissue resulting in inflammation, pain, and often the gradual destruction of joints. There is also an inheritable component to rheumatoid arthritis; if a family member had it, you are more likely to get it.

Osteoarthritis is the more common form of arthritis. More than 80% of individuals older than fifty-five have evidence of osteoarthritis on X-rays with the hips and knees being the joints most often affected. Osteoarthritis can be thought of as a sort of "wear and tear" arthritis usually due to repetitive trauma and the gradual breakdown of joint tissue with age.

Unfortunately, most of us do have some degree of osteoarthritis or will develop it as we grow older. But there are things we can do to help prevent it if we don't have it and to limit and curtail its progression if we do.

> If you have arthritis, staying strong, flexible, aligned, and active can help limit pain and prevent progression.

> If you don't have arthritis, staying strong, flexible, aligned, and active can help prevent it.

Cartilage

Cartilage protects our joints. Cartilage is like a living Teflon layer lining the inside of our joints that acts to prevent bone from rubbing directly against bone. Like a water balloon, cartilage also acts to both buffer and distribute forces equally throughout entire joint surfaces so that forces are not concentrated in only one area.

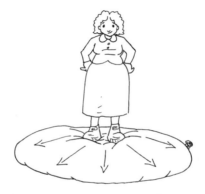

With aging and the repetitive trauma that goes along with it, it is believed that small cracks and tears (microtrauma) occur in cartilage surfaces. This attracts the attention of the body's immune system. Our body perceives these breaks as a threat, and it responds dramatically.

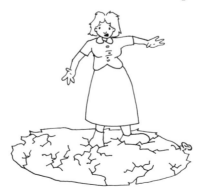

With mal-alignment and with stiff, inflexible joints, we become more prone to developing arthritis. A hip that can't move means that forces will be concentrated in only one section of cartilage and that area will be battered and pounded over and over again. It is as if our woman is standing and jumping up and down on just one area of our water balloon. Eventually something has to give.

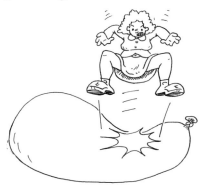

Non-Steroidal Medications

While the non-steroidal, over-the-counter medications (Motrin™, Advil™, Nuprin™, Aleve™, and Naprosyn™) can be life-saving to many, it makes sense to avoid taking them on a chronic basis unless you absolutely have to. Along with other potentially dangerous side-effects, the non-steroidals all actually have adverse effects on the functioning of cartilage cells.

But first, let's clear up one thing—

Anytime a Joint Hurts, It Isn't Arthritis

After a certain age anytime a joint hurts many of us are too quick to label it arthritis. *If your joints hurt consistently, see your doctor,* but pain in joints and the muscles surrounding them can be brought on by any number of things.

> Anytime a joint hurts after a certain age, it isn't arthritis.

Our same three culprits—weakness of muscles, inflexibility, and mal-alignment—can cause pain in our joints and surrounding tissues, pain that may mimic the pain of arthritis.

Pain is a sign that something is off. It can mean that excessive pressure is being put on an area where it shouldn't be. It can mean that our alignment is off, and forces are being concentrated on only one area of a joint. It can mean that certain muscles are weak, and other muscles are protesting at having to do all the work. It can mean that an inflexible muscle is continually being pushed to its limits. Even simply using a joint that hasn't been used in awhile can make it hurt. Left to their own devices, all these things may contribute to arthritis; but early on, they are simply warning signs that something is off.

A great variety of muscle and ligamentous disorders such as bursitis, tendonitis, myositis, and ligamentous strain can mimic the pain of arthritis. All these are fancy words for saying something is off and putting pressure where it shouldn't be, or that some area surrounding a joint is taking excessive punishment.

Discomfort in your joints may even be a sign that you need to do more rather than less. It may mean that something is off and is amenable to change—improved alignment, strengthening, or becoming more flexible.

> Don't be too quick to label any pain in your joints as arthritis and let it curtail your activity. Pain in your joints may be a sign that you need to do more rather than less.

The danger of making too quick of a diagnosis of arthritis for ourselves is that we may relinquish ourselves to having a chronic disease, take to using pain suppressors on a chronic basis, and not do the things that may correct the problem. By doing less, we may make things worse. Instead of doing things that may correct the problem, we may be guaranteeing the persistence and progression of the problem.

Preventing Arthritis

Just as with heart disease and many other disorders, there can be a long lapse of time where damage is occurring to a part of the body but it is not yet clinically evident. It is the same with arthritis. There can be a long period of time where damage is occurring to our joints but it has not yet gotten bad enough to become painful or to show on an X-ray. You may be damaging your joints and not yet know it. Or you may be not doing things that could prevent arthritis.

> What we are doing, or not doing, now may be setting the stage for arthritis later.

Here are the things that affect joint health and what we can do about them. First, there are certain things with regard to our joint health that we can't change. We can't change our genetics (race, sex, body build, family history). We can't change the activity level or nutritional status we had as children (both of which affect joint health), nor any past history of injury or repetitive trauma.

But there are a number of things we can alter that contribute to our joint health. I may be sounding like a broken record by now, but they are same things talked about throughout this book.

Strength: The strength of the muscles surrounding a joint. Our joints are supported by our muscles, and their movement is modulated and controlled by the strength of the muscles surrounding them. When we walk or move, muscles provide shock-absorbing qualities, which attenuate impact on the joints themselves. Weak muscles, in effect, allow a relative collapse of joint spaces. Joints aren't held in "alert" or "ready" positions but rather slouch down on themselves, setting the stage for damage.

Weakness of quadriceps and hamstring muscles in particular put one at risk for arthritis in the hips and knees.

Flexibility: To the extent that we maximize and maintain our joints' full range of motion, we contribute to their health. Movement throughout its range of motion keeps a joint lubricated and operational. Ligaments and tendons surrounding a joint can become glued together from lack of use. The bones in a joint itself can even fuse or become "frozen" in position from lack of use. Relatively immobile joints are a set-up for arthritis.

Posture: Our joints are designed to carry our weight with specific alignment. When the posture of an individual joint is off, force isn't equally distributed and we risk injury and increased wear and tear. Our body works as a concerted whole. The strength, flexibility, and alignment of the rest of the body affect any given part of the body. If one part isn't doing its job, another area often has to take up the slack. Faulty alignment in one area by definition leads to faulty alignment and compensation somewhere else. Our joints pay the price.

Weight: As if there weren't already enough reasons to lose weight, increased weight increases compression and wear and tear on joints. Excessive weight can potentially increase your chance of developing arthritis is you don't have it yet.

For most of us, unless we are exceptionally strong, if we carry 50 pounds of extra weight around with us wherever you go, it *will* cause more wear and tear on our major weight-carrying joints, primarily our knees and hips. There is no substitute to losing weight if you are overweight and want to protect and preserve your joints.

Activity: Inactivity can contribute to arthritis. Running, skiing, and other repetitive load-bearing sports often get a bad rap as being damaging to our joints. They aren't necessarily damaging to our joints, but they are damaging to our joints when we do them *without* adequate strength, flexibility, alignment, and technique.

> By getting and staying strong, by increasing and maintaining the flexibility of your joints, by aligning your body, keeping your weight down and staying active, you may be able to prevent arthritis or at least mitigate its effects.

And Even If You Do Have Arthritis

And even if you do have bona fide arthritis as diagnosed by your physician, proper exercise may drastically ease the symptoms and prevent or slow the progression of the disease. Weight loss (if you are overweight) can also decrease the symptoms of arthritis and slow its progression.

Talk to your doctor. Current treatment of arthritis includes staying active and preserving and maintaining muscle strength and joint flexibility.

The general rule is that no strengthening or stretching exercise should cause severe pain at the time of the exercise or lasting more than two hours after finishing. Neither should there be increased joint inflammation or excessive pain on the day following the exercise regimen.

No matter what our limitations, there is always something we can do. Remember, often a little activity can make a big difference. There are so many variations on exercises available that you can always find some variation that works for you. There is always an exercise that can maintain the strength of the muscles surrounding any given joint. Talk to your doctor or physical therapist. Look at exercise books.

> Find a series of exercises that work for you no matter what your limitations.

> **Change The Way You Think:** By getting and staying strong, flexible, and aligned we can prevent arthritis or limit its progression.

Let's take a look at another common malady—back pain ...

Suggested Resources

Strong Women and Men Beat Arthritis: The Scientifically Proven Program That Allows People With Arthritis to Take Charge of Their Disease, Miriam Nelson, PhD et al, Perigee Books, 2003. I heartily recommend all of Dr. Nelson's "Strong" series of books. Among other things, she encourages and provides simple strengthening exercises beneficial to all of us.

Wear and Tear: Stop the Pain and Put the Spring Back in Your Body,,Bob Arnot and Robert Burns Arnot; Simon & Schuster, 2002. An informative book that reviews much of the current literature of muscle and joint health.

CHAPTER 12

Back Pain

*If your spine is stiff and inflexible
at thirty, you are old. If your spine
is flexible at sixty, you are young.*

—Joseph Pilates

If there is one area of our body that many of us believe is suspect, it is our back. Whether we blame it on walking upright, a genetic predisposition ("My dad had a bad back, you know"), the demands of our occupation, or simply a major flaw in the design of our bodies, the facts are sobering.

Millions of people are incapacitated by back pain every year causing billions of dollars in direct and indirect costs. At any given time, it is estimated that one in eight people is suffering from back pain.

Anyone who has had back pain—and after a certain age, that apparently means most of us—knows how incapacitating it can be. Paroxysms of pain can leave us clutching the sides of our bed or unable to maneuver ourselves in or out of our cars. Chronic back pain can dominate our days usurping huge chunks of our time and energy and severely limiting what we can or cannot do.

> Much back pain can be remedied and prevented by getting and staying strong, flexible, and aligned.

The Straw That Broke The Camel's Back

Back problems seemingly occur out of the blue—a sudden twist, lifting something we are unaccustomed to, or a particularly vigorous warrior weekend. But one common theme in this book is that, while pain or injury in our joints or muscles may occur as acute events, underlying weakness, stiffness, and mal-alignment often set the stage for this to occur. And that includes problems with our back.

> Many of our muscle and joint pains and injuries seem to occur out to the blue, but underlying deterioration in our strength, flexibility, and alignment are often what contribute to them happening.

The straw that breaks the camels' back—in this case, our back—may have been a long time coming.

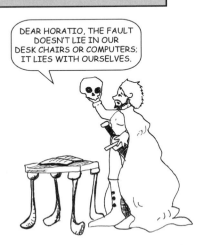

And there is not a problem with our chairs or computers that causes our back pain. If our backs are strong and flexible, we should be able to sit and work in a variety of environments without problems. Our mattresses have enough coiled springs per square inch.

The Spinal Column Is Not Really A Column

Not like the ones that make up the Parthenon or the great temples in ancient Rome. A true column supports the weight of a structure. Our spinal column is a semi-flexible structure supported by muscles and ligaments, which stretch out from it much the way guy lines suspend and support a tent pole.

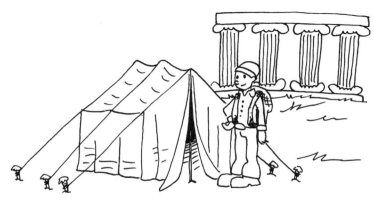

It is the muscles and ligaments that surround our
spine that support it and give it lift.

The muscles that support our back lie in several layers along the sides of our spine. It is often the deeper layers that aren't readily apparent that become weak first. And it takes exercise that we don't usually get in our daily lives to strengthen these muscles and keep them strong. The muscles on the front and sides of our trunk complement these back muscles. It is

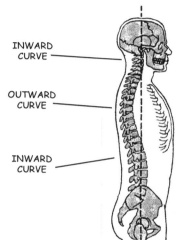

INWARD
CURVE

OUTWARD
CURVE

INWARD
CURVE

both the strength and the balance between these opposing muscle groups that create optimal spine support.

All these muscles also act as shock absorbers buffeting and attenuating the forces on our spine. When our muscles are weak, those forces are more likely to be transmitted directly to our ligaments, bones, and discs.

The spinal column is optimally designed to carry our weight with a gentle S-shaped curve. There is a slight inward (concave) curve at our neck, an outward (convex) curve at our thoracic back, and another deeper inward curve in our low back. These curves are important. Alterations in these curves, such as too much arch or too little arch in the low back, allow forces to be disproportionately concentrated where they shouldn't be.

An ingenious design of small blocks (vertebrae) separated by gelatinous squashed balls (discs) enable flexibility and balance the forces carried up and down the spine. However, the discs—so often seemingly the guilty parties—really don't or shouldn't carry much weight; the weight that they *do* carry should be evenly distributed both throughout the spine and evenly throughout the surface of each disc. Each individual disc should carry its fair share of the load and, ideally, weight should be evenly distributed throughout the surface area of each disc.

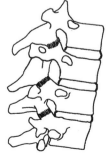

What Causes Back Pain?

Lots of things. A great number of medical conditions, many of them quite serious, can cause back pain: kidney infections, kidney stones, ulcers, tumors, aortic aneurysms, and others. *See your doctor.* This book isn't designed to be a comprehensive guide to the diagnosis and treatment of back pain.

> The signs of a herniated disc putting pressure on a nerve root are any of the following: leg pain, numbness or loss of sensation in your lower extremities, weakness of muscles in your legs, or any bladder problems. These are all signs you need to see your doctor right away.

Sciatica is the general term for irritation of the sciatic nerve, the largest nerve in the body. Nerve roots from the spinal cord intermingle to form the sciatic nerve (one on each side), which then runs deep in the buttocks and down the thigh before branching out in the calf and foot. Irritation or compression of the sciatic nerve anywhere from its origin to its final destination can cause pain.

A herniated disc in the low back puts pressure on the nerve roots that form the sciatic nerve. Hence, classic pain from a herniated disc radiates from the low back on the side of or behind the thigh often extending all the way down the leg into the calf muscles and foot. In older individuals, a narrowing of the spinal canal, termed spinal stenosis and often caused by arthritic changes, can also put pressure on the nerve roots causing sciatica.

That said, most back pain is not caused by a herniated disc. Most back pain is caused by stretching or tearing of muscles or ligaments, or underused muscles going into spasm. And our same three culprits—weakness, stiffness, and mal-alignment—cause or contribute to much back pain. Here's how—

- We twist in a way we aren't accustomed to or lift something heavier than we are used to. An inflexible muscle is suddenly called upon to do its duty. It is forced to be stretched beyond its limits. Microtears occur in the muscle. This causes pain. Other muscles contract and go into spasm to protect or splint that area.

- We are required to lift something heavy. The muscles in our legs, back, and abdomen are weak. Weak, under-utilized muscles go into spasm like a seatbelt locking up when pulled on suddenly. Or if our muscles can't support the weight, it is transmitted to ligaments and discs straining and damaging them. Correct lifting mechanics (bending your knees, etc.) allow us to maximize the strength that we have in the muscles that are *most normally* strong. But if those muscles are weak also, we are still at risk.

- Alterations in our posture concentrate forces in one area of our spine or low back. Certain muscles work overtime while others skate by. Over time those muscles carrying the brunt of the load become frazzled and weary and go into spasm.

- Weight gain increases the load our spine needs to carry. The effects of any alterations in posture are magnified.

Any and all of these can lead to back pain.

The general rule for acute back pain is to rest—but not too long. Let pain be your guide. During the acute event, if it hurts to do something or move a certain way, don't do it. But get up and move as soon as possible. Inactivity breeds further compromise in strength and flexibility. For most people, one or two days of rest are enough.

Disc Disease

As stated above, the great percentage of people with back pain don't have disc disease. And it's curious to note that a fair number of people *without* back pain have bulging, herniated discs on radiological studies.

One of the themes of this book is that the location of a pain may not be its source. Just because you hurt in a certain area doesn't mean it is that area that is causing the pain. The pain could be caused by a problem in the alignment of your shoulders or hips or weak muscles somewhere else that *cause* the pain to be felt there.

> The location of pain is often not its true source.

And the same is true for X-rays or other radiological studies. Just because there are changes on an X-ray in a certain area doesn't necessarily mean that that area is the source of the problem. Remember, our bodies are integrated wholes. The area where bone breaks down on an X-ray often only represents the area where forces are being concentrated enough to cause damage.

> The location of an abnormality on an X-ray is often not the source of the problem.

This often applies to disc disease. A bulging disc on an MRI is more often just the location where altered forces are being concentrated enough to become manifest. The disc is a weak link in the mechanical chain and it bulges and ruptures.

Surgery may remove or immobilize a troublesome disc and alleviate pressure on a nerve. But if we focus solely on the abnormal pathology and attempt only to correct it, we often risk solutions that are palliative at best. The pain is often postponed for a while and comes back later in the same place or somewhere else because the altered forces which created or contributed to the problem to begin with aren't fully remedied.

You remember from Chapter 5 that the alignment of our pelvis in great part influences the curves in our back. A pelvis that is tilted too far forward causes an increased curve in our low back, potentially putting excessive pressure on the front part of the discs.

When our pelvis is tilted backward, we lose the natural curve in our low back. Our low back becomes flatter; this puts excessive pressure on the back of the discs.

> Strengthening and aligning the muscles surrounding our pelvis can help our back.

The Downward Spiral In Back Pain

Back pain is a complicated subject. It would be naïve to suggest that all back pain is solely caused by mal-alignment or weak muscles. But one would be equally remiss not to suggest that these things, if not the cause, at least contribute to a great deal of our back pain.

The same familiar story is often repeated with back pain. A predominantly sedentary lifestyle (lots of sitting) allows weakness and stiffness in key muscle groups, which contribute to faulty alignment. Weakness, stiffness, and faulty alignment put us at risk for back pain. Pain and decreased function limit our activity further. Muscles become weaker and stiffer. We become less active. We gain weight. We learn to live with it or work around the pain. A series of palliative remedies is tried—the pain eventually comes back. And on it goes.

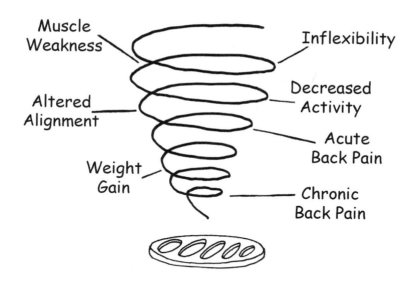

Muscle Weakness — Inflexibility — Decreased Activity — Altered Alignment — Acute Back Pain — Weight Gain — Chronic Back Pain

Staying strong, flexible, and aligned is the best insurance policy against back pain.

How To Bend Without Hurting Yourself

One way to lift is by bending your knees and straightening your legs to stand up. That can help. But a second key point is to lift without allowing your back to go into full flexion, that is, without allowing your low back to round completely. Instead we want to keep our back braced and some curve in our low back. To do this takes core strength.

Try this. Stand several feet away from a table or countertop. Bend forward at your waist and place your hands on the surface of the table. Now, purposely put a small arch in your low back, and lift up to standing using your back and abdominal muscles without loosing the arch in your back. Can you do it? Your belly and your back muscles will have to do the work.

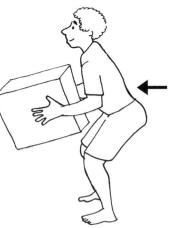

While I don't recommend lifting in an extended position like this, having the awareness to keep some arch in your back and not allowing it to go into full forward tilt is a key to safe lifting.

Why Don't Back Exercises Work

Because we don't do them enough. We don't do them hard enough or long enough. Many of us are big, stiff, weak, and crooked. We often have big, bulky bodies with tight muscles that hold us in contracted positions. It's going to take more than five minutes of exercise once a day to realign and strengthen key muscle groups in our back.

Back Exercises

Here are back exercises useful to preserving and maintaining a healthy back. Their goal is to maintain healthy flexibility (forward, backward, and to the sides), strength, and alignment. Do them in order.

1. Table Stretch
Page 185

8. Bridge
Page 165

2. Standing Side
Stretch
Page 184

9. Floor Twist
Page 172

3. Couch Stretch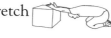
Page 168

10. Abdominal
Crunches
Page 162

4. Cats and Dogs
Page 165

11. Side Crunches
Page 180

5. Downward Dog
Page 169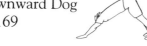

12. Cobra
Page 167

6. Child's Pose
Page 166

13. Bow
Page 165

7. Hamstring Stretch
with Strap
Page 173

14. Locust
Page 177

continued on next page

15. Standing Bent-Knee
Chair Twist
Page 183

17. Wall Bench
Page 188

16. Forward Bend
at Wall
Page 172

18. Astronaut
Page 163

Change The Way You Think: Our backs are reliable structures *if* we stay strong, flexible, and aligned. We can do something ourselves to remedy much of our back pain.

The next chapter contains detailed descriptions of all the exercises used throughout this book ...

CHAPTER 13

Exercises

Exercise strengthens and inactivity wastes.

—Hippocrates

For convenience, all of the exercises in this book are described in detail in this single chapter. Many of the same exercises are prescribed repeatedly for different problems throughout the book. That is because many of our problems share common deficits in strength, flexibility, and alignment. All of the exercises are carefully chosen. They work.

Read the instructions closely. Some of the exercises may sound like exercises you have done before, but there are usually a few variations that make them more effective. After doing an exercise for several days, it is usually a good idea to go back and reread the instructions. There are often things you may have missed or didn't make sense until you have done the exercise for a while.

Some of the exercises may be harder than what you are used to. Exercises that are too easy won't restore or maintain our muscles and joints. Challenge yourself. Use your own judgment on what is best for you, but consider the fact that in most cases we need and can do more than we think. Also, it is the *trying* that builds the strength, flexibility, and coordination we need.

In many of the exercise menus throughout the book, the exercises are prescribed in a specific numbered sequence. Exercises that allow you to warm up a little are first, while more demanding exercises are later in the sequences. Also, the menus of exercises are designed to systematically work on a problem. Stretching one area *first* often allows another area to stretch or align itself. By doing the exercises in order, you will get maximum benefit.

Some of the other exercise menus (not numbered) are more like a smorgasbord for a given area of the body. Choose one or more of those exercises to address that specific area or problem. Or add them to your current exercise program.

I encourage you to try all the exercises listed below over a period of time. Find the ones that work for you. Add and subtract exercises as your ability improves.

A few more tips—

- Make sure you do the exercises with correct alignment. We want to reinforce and strengthen correct posture and body alignment every time we exercise. Correct alignment unless stated otherwise includes—

  - Feet pointing straight ahead. Feet hip-width apart.

  - Hips level. One hip shouldn't be more forward or lifted more than the other. Be aware of this also in the supine (lying on your back) exercises; one hip shouldn't be cocked higher than the other.

  - Shoulders back. A good way to remember this is to consciously lift your shoulders up, then back, and then relax them down.

  - Low back in neutral. This means you want some curve in your low back; you don't want it completely flat nor do you want it excessively arched.

- Get a small timer. That way you can accurately time how long you are holding each exercise and over time increase it. Without a timer, you end up guessing or looking at a clock.

- A yoga mat or a carpeted area works best for doing most of these exercises.

- Do the exercises barefoot if possible. Give your feet a workout too. Many of the exercises specifically address muscles in our feet and calves; for them you need bare feet.

- For the strengthening exercises, make sure you hold yourself up long enough or do enough reps until the muscles that are being addressed get fatigued. That is what builds strength (remember Chapter 7). The amount of time and the number of reps are approximations; do the number of reps or hold the exercise for long enough so that it fatigues *your* muscles. This is different for each person. Increase the reps and the amount of time as you grow stronger.

- Breathe. Don't hold your breath while exercising. Straining and holding your breath while exercising can actually cause your heart rate to precipitously drop. The general rule for breathing while exercising is to exhale on the contractile portion of an exercise, that is, when you are lifting a weight or straining, and to inhale on the relaxation portion, when you release the weight down. For flexibility exercises, the general rule is to exhale as you bend forward or close the body in on itself, and inhale as you stretch upward or bend backward. Breathe.

- Relax the parts that aren't doing the work. Don't scrunch up your face and neck.

- For the flexibility or stretching exercises, once you are familiar with the exercise, make sure you stretch close to your limits. Don't just go through the motion. Use caution but really stretch (see Chapter 8).

- How often should you do the exercises? Every other day would be great.

Dumbing Down

Too often for older individuals (again, whatever age you pick), there is a dumbing down of exercise. Exercises are made so simple and undemanding as to be almost inconsequential. In advertisements the older individual is seen as someone so helpless as to be gleeful to just lift their arms above their head.

While I recognize that there are infirm or incapacitated individuals for whom many of these types of exercises are helpful, for most of us they aren't enough. In fact, if we aren't careful, they put us at risk for a self-fulfilling spiral where demanding less of ourselves makes us able to do less.

That's why many of the exercises in this book are demanding. If you are going to spend the time doing something, get the maximum benefit from it by doing something hard and challenging. If you are going to take an exercise class, take the one with the twenty-year olds. Don't lift weights far below your threshold; don't stretch well within your limits.

> Run with the big dogs.

List Of Exercises

Ab Stretch

A large exercise ball works best for this. Lie backward over the exercise ball. If you are new to using one of these balls, be careful. It takes a 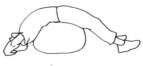 little while to adjust your balance. If you roll your shoulders over the ball, you get a nice stretch in your shoulders. But instead, roll farther down on the ball so that your abdomen and bottom are arched over the ball. You should feel a stretch across your belly and groin. Relax. Let go. Do this for fifteen seconds or longer.

Abdominal Crunches

Lie on your back with your feet against a wall with your knees and legs forming a ninety-degree angle with the rest of your body. Lift your arms above your head with your elbows slightly bent. Now 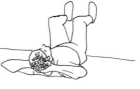 lift your head, neck, arms, and shoulders *upward* toward the ceiling. Your head and neck only need to come off the floor about six inches. You want to lift upward, not forward toward your toes. Hold for a second and relax completely back down.

Do twenty, gradually working your way up to fifty over time.

Once you get the hang of this, try doing this without the wall, that is, with your legs still at ninety degrees and suspended in the air. Or as another variation, hold an exercise ball or several pillows up between your knees while you do your crunches.

Airplane

Lie on your stomach with your legs stretched out and your feet pigeon-toed so that your big toes touch. Extend your arms out to the sides at shoulder level with your palms facing 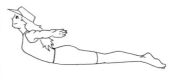 downward. Now, in one controlled motion, lift your head, shoulders, upper back, and arms off the floor. Try to initiate the movement from your tailbone region. Once you are up, focus on lifting your arms in an up-and-backward direction. You are now cleared for takeoff.

Hold for fifteen seconds, rest for a few seconds and repeat. If this is too difficult, try locking your feet underneath a couch or similar object for added support, then over time work your way up to the full posture.

Arm Circles

Stand with your feet hip-width apart. Lift your arms out to the sides, shoulder high. Relax your shoulders so that they are not hunched up around your neck. Your arms should be straight and level.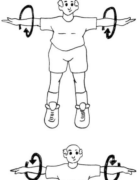

With your thumbs pointing forward make thirty small circles (ten inches in diameter) in the forward direction. Then point your thumbs backward and your palms up and do thirty circles in the reverse direction. Strive to open up your chest and push your shoulders back without letting them rise up around your ears.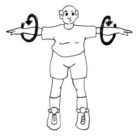

Once you get used to doing the small circles, try doing a set maximizing the rotation of your arms. Everything else remains the same except on the forward circles tilt your hands so that they are facing backward (the backs of your hands face forward) and you feel the stretch in a different area of your shoulders. For the backward circles, exaggerate the tilt of your hands backward.

Astronaut

Lie on your back with your bent legs resting on a couch, chair, bed, or ottoman. Take some time to find or make something the correct height—not too high or too low—so that your body can form a ninety-degree angle, and your legs are 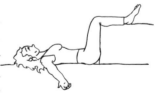 supported and can rest comfortably on top. Your arms are at your sides, palms up. Make sure your seat is not too far away from whatever you are using. Now relax. Let your pelvis and your lower back relax into the floor. Don't force them or try to make this happen; this is a gravity exercise.

Give this exercise at least five minutes to do its thing. Ten minutes would be even better.

My sister calls this exercise the "Astronaut" because the positioning approximates that of an astronaut in an early space capsule: "Apollo Five, this is Houston ... can you read me?"

Back Stretch

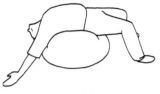

This one feels so good. The purchase of a large exercise ball is worth it just to do this exercise. If you haven't used one of these balls before, be careful at first. It takes a few tries to figure out your balance.

Lie backward over the ball allowing your chest and shoulders to open downward. Tell yourself to relax. Allow gravity to do the work.

Experiment with your positioning on the ball. The farther forward you are on the ball, the more it stretches your shoulders and upper back—both good things. By positioning your buttocks more on the ball, the front of your groin and pelvis are stretched. Try and keep your feet hip-width apart and pointing straight backward. Relax and feel the stretch.

If you don't have an exercise ball, lie off the edge of a bed allowing your shoulders and upper back to relax downward.

Boat

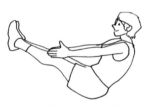

Sit on the floor with you legs extended out in front of you. Now lift your legs off the floor and extend them upward at about a forty-five degree angle as you tilt your body backward also at about a forty-five degree angle. Try to keep your weight centered on the upper part of your buttocks. *Keep your back straight and lifted with a slight arch in it; don't let it sag backward.* Your arms extend out in front of you parallel to the floor with your palms facing toward each other. If this is too difficult, bend your knees slightly and hold on with your hands behind your knees. Don't compromise your form, that is, don't let your back sag.

After fifteen seconds turn your upper body and your arms toward the right and hold for another fifteen seconds. Then return to center and turn toward the left and hold.

As you improve, increase the time spent in each position. The key to doing this exercise is to only do it as long as you can keep a slight arch in your back without your back sagging backward.

Bow

Lie on your stomach. Your chin rests on the floor. Bend your knees, reach backward, and grab the outside of your feet with your hands. In one smooth motion, lift your chest, thighs, and legs upward so that you are balanced on your pelvis. *Lift toward*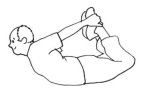
the ceiling. Try to keep your knees hip-width apart or pulled toward each other; don't let them flare out to the side. Focus on opening your shoulders backward and lifting your thighs off the ground as well. Breathe. Hold for ten seconds, relax down and rest, and then repeat. Work on feeling the stretch symmetrically throughout the entire length of your back.

Bridge

This is a challenging exercise that strengthens the back and glute muscles. Lie on your back with your knees bent and your feet flat on the floor, hip-width apart, and pointing straight ahead. Your hands should rest comfortably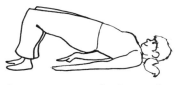
at your sides, palms down. Make sure your body is in a straight line, that is, you don't want to be cocked to one side or the other. Lift your bottom straight up off the floor toward the ceiling. Your weight remains supported by your head, shoulders, arms, and the bottoms of your feet. Keep your neck straight; don't let it turn to either side. Lift as high as you can toward the ceiling. Don't just go through the motions; try to get that extra push upward at the top. You should feel this in your buttocks and in your low back. Hold for ten to fifteen seconds and then lower your bottom slowly back down toward the floor. Repeat.

Cats and Dogs

Get down on your hands and knees so that your back forms a small table. Your hands should be directly below your shoulders with your fingers pointing forward. Your knees should be directly below your hips, forming a right angle. Now, exhale and arch your back upward like a cat. Do this slowly and consciously making sure you focus on curving your neck (chin toward chest), your upper back, your lower back, and your pelvis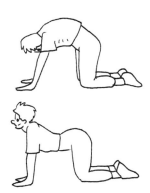

so that you form one smooth curve with the back of your body. *Focus particularly on getting the last few degrees of tilt to your pelvis.*

Hold for a few seconds then slowly arch in the other direction. While keeping your hands and knees where they are, arch your head and neck upward, your upper and lower back downward, and lift your buttocks into the air, opening them outward. Again, try to make sure you get the last few degrees of tilt to your pelvis so that you feel it in your groins. This is the dog stretch.

Hold for a few seconds and then smoothly transition to the cat stretch. Repeat ten cycles.

Chair Twist

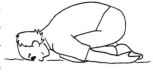

For this exercise you will need a chair with a firm bottom, a back, and no arms. A normal kitchen chair or firm office chair works fine. Sit sideways with the right side of your body against the back of the chair. Your feet are hip-width apart and pointing straight ahead. Your weight is evenly balanced on both sitting bones. Now turn your upper body so that the front of your body faces toward the back of the chair; grasp the back portion of the chair to help twist yourself. You should feel the twist in your hips and your upper shoulders and back. Keep your body upright and your shoulders level. Don't let yourself sag. Focus on twisting your upper body.

Hold for thirty seconds. Repeat on the opposite side.

Child's Pose

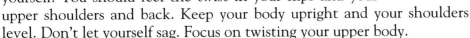

This is a classic yoga relaxation pose, but initially it might not feel so relaxing if your lower back and hamstrings are tight. Sit on the floor Japanese style with your knees bent and your legs underneath you so that you are sitting on your heels. Try to keep both thighs pointing straight ahead. If this is terribly uncomfortable, you can modify the position by putting a small pillow under your bottom. If it is painful for your feet, put a small towel under your feet. Often we are tight in these areas, and it takes time for them to stretch out. Now, roll your body forward so that your chest is on or close to your thighs. Allow your hands to relax down at your sides. Your forehead rests gently on the floor. If your forehead can't touch the floor, you can use another small pillow to support it. You don't want it dangling in the air and causing more tension in your neck and back.

Stay in this position for thirty seconds to one minute or longer. Relax.

Child's Pose on Chair

Sit upright on a hard-bottomed chair. Your feet should be shoulder-width apart and pointing straight ahead. Place a pillow or cushion on your lap. Now, allow your upper body to fold and relax forward so that your chest lies on the pillow close to your thighs. Let your head, shoulders, and arms droop forward. You want to relax and let go in 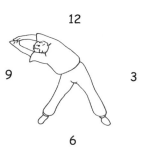 this pose, so make sure you have the right sized pillow. No tension; no holding on.

Relax in this pose for thirty seconds to one minute.

Clock

Stand with your feet three and one half feet apart. Lift both arms above your head, keeping your palms facing forward and interlocking your thumbs. This is twelve o'clock. Now slowly rotate your torso and arms to the right, for the upper numbers of the clock keeping your arms as close to the same plane as your body as you can. Don't fold forward and try to keep your shoulders opening outward. Proceed slowly around the clock until you are hanging completely downward at six o'clock. Relax for a few seconds and then continue around until once again your arms are pointing upward at twelve o'clock. Go slowly. Stay in control. You should feel this in your flanks and on the sides of your body.

Go around the clock three times in the forward direction and then three times in reverse. Then it's time to quit.

Cobra

Lie on your stomach with your feet pigeon-toed (pointing inward) so that your big toes touch. Your forehead is touching the floor. Place your hands under your shoulders so that the tips of your fingers

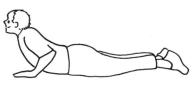

are at the level of the tops of your shoulders. Keep your elbows in. Now, while pressing your thighs and pelvis into the floor, lift your head, neck, shoulders, and upper back off the floor using the strength of your upper back. Your head and neck arch slightly backward; don't overly tense them or scrunch them up around your ears. You should only rise a few inches off the floor. No weight should be carried by your hands; they are simply there for balance. Try to bring your shoulders slightly back and toward each other so that you feel a slight pinch between your shoulder blades.

Hold for ten seconds, rest, and then repeat.

Couch Stretch

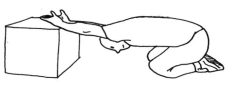

Here's an exercise you can do on the couch! Well, sorta. Kneel down about one and one half to two feet away from a couch or a similar object. A large exercise ball also works well for this. Your toes point straight back behind you, not out to the sides. Stretch your arms forward, resting them palm down on the cushions of the couch while sliding your bottom backward so that your bottom rests on your heels or close to it. You may have to adjust your position to get it just right. Drop your head and shoulders toward the floor. Relax. You want to feel a stretch in your groins and buttocks along with the area between your shoulder blades. Work on extending your bottom backward toward the wall behind you while stretching your arms forward and at the same time relaxing. Let gravity do the work. One minute is good; two minutes is better.

As a variation, you can try turning your palms upward slightly. This deepens the stretch to the shoulders.

Crossover Hip Stretch

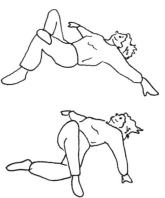

Lie on your back with your knees bent. Make sure that your pelvis is centered and that one hip isn't tilted or out to the side. Cross your right leg so that your right foot rests on your left thigh just above the knee. Next, twist your hips toward the left so that your right foot comes down toward the floor while remaining in contact with your thigh. Concentrate on pushing your right knee away from your body while trying to open up your thigh like a book. You should feel a stretch in your right groin and around your thigh.

Hold and stretch for fifteen to thirty seconds and then repeat on the opposite side.

Deep Squat

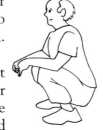

Many people throughout the world spend much of their lives squatting. They squat to prepare meals, to work, to eat, to converse with friends, and to go to the bathroom. Squatting stretches our hips, legs, buttocks, and back.

Squat down. Try to keep your feet pointing straight ahead and hip-width apart. There is a tendency for your feet to want to point outward, but that is not what we want with this. Try to shift your weight backward and if possible allow your feet to be flat on the floor rather than lifted up on your toes. If your Achilles tendons are tight, this will be tough. Listen to your own body and do what you can; at first, you may need to hold onto something in front of you. Focus on pulling your body upward so, instead of leaning forward, your torso is vertical. Open up your chest slightly and let your shoulders relax down and back. Hold for one minute.

If this exercise hurts your knees excessively, don't do it.

Downward Dog

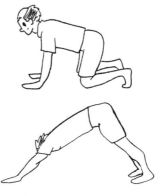

This is a classic yoga pose. Some yoga teachers say that if you do only one yoga exercise, this is the one to do. It stretches out the entire back of the body including the lower back and hamstrings. Get on the floor on your hands and knees. Your hands are directly under your shoulders; your knees are hip-width apart. Now, while leaving your hands and feet where they are, slowly push yourself up, lifting your bottom high in the air so that your body forms a triangle. Your hands are evenly spaced with your fingers pointing forward; your feet are hip-width apart with your toes pointing forward. Your back should be straight, that is, not sagging toward the floor nor overly lifting or arching upward. Ideally, you want your weight evenly balanced between your hands and feet. If you can get your heels to the ground, that's great; if not, don't worry about it but keep your feet pointing straight ahead. Focus on lifting your bottom *up* and *back*.

Hold for fifteen to thirty seconds.

If you can't do the whole pose, that's okay. Instead, just get down on your hands and knees (with feet and hands pointing straight ahead) and push up in any manner so that your weight is on your hands and feet. Don't worry initially about how straight your back is. Just get the feel of supporting yourself on your hands and feet. Doing this even for a few seconds begins to strengthen muscles and provides a needed stretch to the back of your body.

Elbow Curls

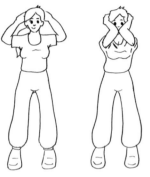

Stand with your feet hip-width apart and pointing straight ahead. Bend your elbows and touch the tips of your fingers to your temples just above your ears. Your elbows should be splayed out like wings. Open them up as wide as you can while keeping your fingers in contact with your temples. Now move both elbows forward—keeping your fingers in contact with your temples—while trying to get your elbows to meet in front of your face. *Stretch* to make your elbows meet. Then pull your elbows back, remembering to bring them as far back as possible while keeping your fingers in contact with your temples.

That's one. Do twenty of these.

Face Plant

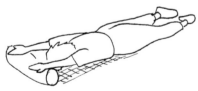

Lie on your stomach with a large firm pillow about eight inches high at arms length above your head. A couch cushion works fine. Extend your legs straight backward and turn your feet inward (pigeon-toed) so that your big toes just touch. Extend your arms palms upward above your head so that they rest on the pillow and are shoulder-width apart. Your face rests on the floor with your nose and chin touching the floor and not tilted up or to either side—hence the name of the exercise. Relax. The idea is to allow gravity to begin to relax the tight muscles around your shoulders and upper back. Give this exercise time to work; I know at first it may be uncomfortable. After a few seconds you should begin to feel this in the backs of your shoulders as they begin to let go.

Hold for two minutes, working up to five minutes.

Face the Wall

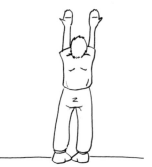

Stand facing a wall with your feet hip-width apart and your toes turned inward and touching (pigeon-toed). Your chest and nose should be close to the wall. Lift your arms straight above your head and place them on the wall, turning your hands inward so that your little fingers are turned toward each other. This may be tough at first. Try to let your shoulders relax; don't keep them bunched up around your ears.

Hold this position for one minute (use your timer), working your way up to three minutes. Concentrate on maintaining your hip and foot position and on turning your arms inward. You should feel this in the backs of your shoulders and your groin.

Floor Sit

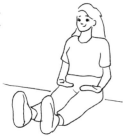

Find a comfortable wall. Sit down on the floor with your seat pressed up against the wall. Extend your legs, keeping your legs together and your toes pointing toward the ceiling. You don't have to hold your feet or ankles flexed, but you don't want them rolling out to either side. Your bottom, the backs of your shoulders, and your head touch the wall. If your shoulders are normally rolled forward, this may be difficult at first. Do the best you can, over time working toward correct positioning. Turn your hands palm up, fingers pointing toward the middle, and place them on your upper thighs. This helps to ensure that your shoulders remain positioned back against the wall. Relax. Are your legs still aligned and your toes still pointing upward? Do you feel the weight evenly distributed on both of your sitting bones? You should feel this exercise in your shoulders, the front of your chest, and also often in your groin region and lower back—everywhere.

Hold this position for two to three minutes or longer.

Floor Twist

Lie on the floor on your right side with your 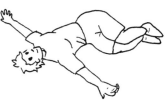 knees forming a ninety-degree angle. Your arms are out to the right, one on top of the other in line with your shoulders. While leaving your knees in place, slowly rotate your upper (left) arm and shoulder upward and across to your left side. You should feel this in your left hip and shoulder. The idea is to, over time, get your left shoulder and arm to lie flat on the floor while keeping your knees in position. Go slow and be gentle with this—listen to your body. You may place a pillow under your left shoulder or arm if you are particularly stiff to begin with. Pressing down gently on your right knee with your right hand accentuates the stretch. Over time, attempt to turn your head so that it looks away from the bent-knee side.

Hold for one minute. Repeat on the other side.

Bringing your knees up tighter and higher (closer to your arms) makes this exercise more demanding. Stretching out your knees slightly and bringing them downward toward your feet makes it easier. Adjust the position so you feel a stretch appropriate to your level of flexibility.

Make sure that your body remains symmetrically aligned. Even though your hips are twisting, they should not be jutted out to the side. Your arms should remain level with your shoulders on both sides. When you are in the full position, focus on extending and lengthening your uppermost arm away from your body.

Forward Bend at Wall

Stand facing backward to a wall with your feet about ten inches away. Lean back slightly so that your bottom rests against the wall. Straighten your legs, making sure your feet are hip-width apart and pointing straight ahead. Bend forward at the waist. Grasp your elbows with opposite hands and hang. Relax. While keeping your knees straight, let the weight of your body stretch your lower back and your hamstrings. Focus on keeping a small amount of arch in your low back, that is, your bottom moves backward toward the wall while your upper body extends and drops forward. You may also place a small block on the floor, reach down, and hold onto that.

Stretch for thirty seconds.

Groin Stretch

Tight muscles in our groins and low back are reluctant to give up their hold on our bodies. This exercise sneaks up on them using gravity to do the work. For this exercise you need something like a chair, a sofa, a bed, an 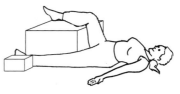 ottoman, or even a coffee table. Take your time and find something the correct height for you. You want something neither too high nor too low so that, when you lie on the floor on your back, one leg can be supported and rest on top of your "platform" forming approximately a ninety-degree angle.

Lie on the floor on your back, bend one leg, and place it on top of whatever you've chosen to use. Stretch the other leg out alongside the object. Make sure your torso is in line with your hips and not cocked to one side. Your bottom should be up close to whatever you are using— almost as if you were sitting in a chair and fell over backward. The toes on the straight leg, that is, the foot alongside the object, should be gently pointing toward the ceiling, not falling to one side or the other. Use a few pillows or a block of some kind to keep your straight-leg foot from falling out to the side. It is less crucial if your bent leg foot rolls outward slightly. Your arms are at your sides with your palms facing up. Relax. This is a passive exercise where you allow gravity to do the work. Over time and by degrees, you will begin to feel the deep muscles in your groins begin to relax and let go.

Rest in this pose for five minutes, and then switch sides. Make sure you do both sides. Ten minutes or more on each side would be even better.

Hamstring Stretch with Strap

For this exercise you need a belt, towel, or strap—anything readily available will do, but a yoga strap works best. Lie on your back with your knees bent and your feet on the floor. Make sure your hips are level; your weight should feel equal on both sides and neither hip should be shifted

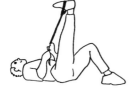 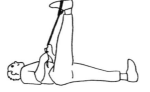 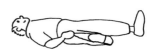

laterally. Lift your right leg and place the strap around the ball of your foot. Straighten the leg, flexing your toes toward you while making sure your foot remains straight in line with your knee and doesn't flare out to the side. Adjust the strap length so that you feel the stretch in your calf muscles and hamstrings. Don't let your hips and shoulders lift off the floor and keep only a small arch in your back (don't absorb the stretch by arching your back too much).

Hold for fifteen seconds and then straighten your left leg (the leg without the strap) so that it is now flat on the floor. Adjust the strap (making it longer) to keep your right leg straight. Hold and stretch for another fifteen seconds. You will feel some of the stretch in your opposite groin; make sure you keep your opposite leg (left) straight as well and don't let it roll out to the side.

Finally, stretch your right leg outward along the floor as high up toward your head as possible. Only stretch as far as you can while keeping your leg straight and maintaining correct alignment. You should feel this in your right groin and a different area of your calf and hamstrings. Stretch for fifteen seconds. Repeat on the other side.

Imaginary Chair

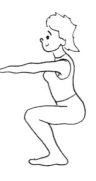

Stand with your feet hip-width apart and your toes pointing straight ahead. Extend your arms out in front of you at shoulder level with your palms down. Now slowly lower yourself down, bending your knees and using your thigh muscles as if you were sitting down on an imaginary chair. Keep your back straight. Try not to bend forward. Try to keep your weight toward your heels. The lower you go, the more demanding it is on your thigh muscles. Challenge yourself without compromising your form or alignment.

Hold for fifteen seconds; over time, work up to a full minute. Then rest for a few seconds and repeat, holding the pose for half as long as you did the first time.

As a variation, you can try doing this exercise while standing on your toes. Everything else remains the same.

Japanese Sitting Pose—Quad Stretch

This sitting pose helps align the spine while stretching the hips and quadriceps muscles. There is a great amount of variation in people's ability to do this, so you have to be willing to adjust the position to find a variation that works for you.

Sit down on the floor Japanese-style with your legs bent underneath you so that you are sitting on your heels and your thighs are together with your knees pointing straight ahead. It is important that your toes point straight back or toward the middle and are not flared open to the sides, which puts a strain on the knees. You should feel the stretch in the tops of your thighs. Keep your upper body vertical; don't lean.

Sit for two minutes.

If this terribly painful to the tops of your feet, put some padding under your feet or place a small cushion or folded blanket under your bottom to ease some of the pressure on them. It also helps to grab the tops of both calf muscles from behind just below your knees and pull them down and to the sides to take some of the strain off your knees.

Once you have mastered the basic pose, you can start to lean backward. Place your hands behind you and start to lean backward. With time, you may be able to settle back on your elbows or even all the way down on your back. Be careful. If this is too painful on your knees, go back to the basic pose. The important thing is to find a variation of this exercise that stretches the front of your thighs *for you*. Listen to your body and don't overdo.

Leg Flop

Lie on your back with your knees bent hip-width apart. Make sure your hips are equally in line with your torso and that one hip isn't tilted or out to the side. Now, leaving your feet in that position simply let your legs fall down toward the floor toward the right. Stretch your arms out to the side leaving your shoulders on the floor. You should feel this stretch on the inside and outside of your thighs. For an additional stretch while in this position you may also place your right foot on top of your left knee.

Relax for one minute and then repeat on the other side.

Leg Lifts

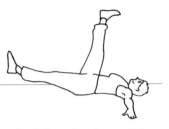

Lie on your back with your legs extended upward at a ninety-degree angle or close to it. Make sure your hips are level and that one isn't cocked to the side more than the other. Flex your feet gently toward your shins. Keeping your left leg extended upward, *slowly* lower your right leg toward the floor. When it is six inches above the floor, pause for a second and then slowly lift it back up. Now repeat, this time dropping your left leg down, holding it, and then lifting. Keep your back and your neck flat against the floor. Don't let them arch. We want our leg and abdominal muscles to do the work. Work your way up to doing ten with each leg.

Now drop both legs down together at the same time. Hover a few inches above the floor and then lift straight up. Work your way up to doing ten of these.

Leg to Chest

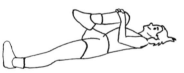

Lie on your back in an aligned position. Bend your right leg and bring it to your chest, wrapping your fingers around your leg several inches below your knee or around your ankle. It helps if you bring your knee slightly outward first before bringing it in and toward your chest. Pull down firmly with your hands to bring your knee as close to your chest as possible. Your head remains flat on the floor. Keep your back flat against the ground—don't let it arch. You should feel a stretch in both groin regions and in your right buttock. Make sure you try to keep your outstretched leg straight (not rolled out to the side), your toes pointing toward the ceiling, and the entire back of your thigh and calf in contact with the floor. Hold and stretch for thirty seconds and then repeat on the opposite side.

Lift-Ups

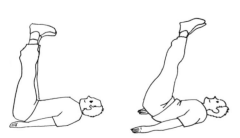

Lie on your back. Make sure your hips are level, that is, that one isn't cocked to the side. Lift your bottom slightly and place your hands palm-side down just under your bottom.

Extend your legs straight up into your air so that they form a ninety-degree angle. Now lift your legs and your bottom straight up into the air several inches toward the ceiling and then relax back down. That's one.

Don't push off from the floor using your hands, but rather try to lift upward using the strength of your abdominal and low back muscles. Try to keep the rest of your body relaxed; don't tense up your shoulders and neck. Breathe. At first, you may only be able to lift an inch or two upward with great effort. That's fine. That means this is a good exercise for you. Try to do five, eventually working your way up to fifteen. Over time work on lifting with a more fluid movement and lifting yourself higher off the floor.

This exercise works the core muscles surrounding our midsection including some of the deeper abdominal muscles which often don't get much of a workout. After doing this exercise for a while along with some of the other core exercises, you should notice yourself standing taller with more lift in your midsection.

Locust

Lie on your stomach with your legs extended hip-width apart and your arms extended forward. Your forehead is touching the 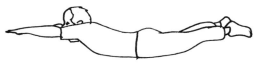 floor. Now, in one controlled movement, lift your head, shoulders, upper back, arms, thighs, and legs off the floor, or as best you can. Try to initiate the movement from your low back region. Relax the muscles in your face or neck. Turn your hands inward slightly, allowing your pinky fingers to come toward each other while keeping your arms shoulder-width apart.

Hold for ten seconds, rest, and then repeat.

Lunge

Find something around two and a half feet high that you can reach out and stretch toward. The arm on a sofa, for example, works fine for this. Stand several paces away and step forward with your right leg, bending your 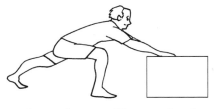 right knee, gently placing your hands on the sofa arm. Your right foot should be pointing straight ahead with your ankle in front of your knee or directly below it, but not behind it. Stay on the toes of your back foot with your foot pointing straight ahead. Focus on keeping your back leg straight. Straightening your back leg while lowering your groin slightly will accentuate the stretch. Is your back foot still pointing straight ahead? Don't let it turn out to the side. Stretch for fifteen seconds, then repeat on the opposite side.

Your strength and flexibility will determine how low you can bend. Pick something the correct height for you. If this is difficult, start by using something higher such as a tabletop.

Lying Side Stretch

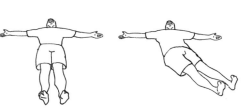

Lie on the floor on your back with your legs outstretched. Make sure your pelvis is centered and not cocked to the side. Now, while leaving your pelvis and upper body in position, slowly slide your feet and legs along the floor to the left while keeping them pointing upward toward the ceiling. Place your left arm above your head on the floor and your left arm at ninety degrees out to the side. If you do this properly, you should feel the stretch along the entire right side of your body. Usually sliding your feet only about a foot is enough. Your feet stay together and your toes point toward the ceiling. Stretch for thirty seconds. Repeat on the opposite side sliding your legs toward the right.

Opposite Arm-Leg

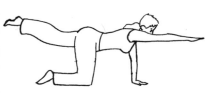

There are multiple benefits to cross-linked movements where one side of our body goes one way and the other goes another. They are great for keeping our neurologic and muscular coordination systems intact and functional. Get down on all fours. Keep your back in neutral. Don't lift it or let it sag down. Extend your right arm directly in front of you while lifting and extending your left leg directly behind you. Focus on creating a consistent line of energy all the way from your right hand across your body and through to your left foot. Gently point and extend your left toes. Hold for a few seconds and then transition to the opposite side, lifting your left arm and right leg. Hold. Repeat five times on each side.

Overhead Stretch

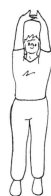

Stand with your feet pointing forward and hip-width apart. Clasp your fingers together and raise them over your head so that your palms point upward. Look upward toward the backs of your hands. Concentrate on trying to get your shoulders up and back, that is, opening them up outward. *Lengthen and extend your body upward.* Ideally, the palms of your hands should be directly overhead so that your entire body, shoulders included, are in one plane.

Hold for thirty seconds, working your way up to a minute.

Pigeon

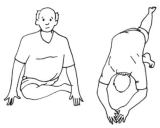

This is a slightly more advanced yoga posture. Come to a deep lunge position with your right foot forward and your left foot lying flat on the floor. Slowly walk your right foot over toward the inside of your body and relax your right leg downward. Your right knee should be outside of your body. Slide and adjust your right foot up toward your head (intensifies the stretch) or down toward your feet to get the right stretch for you. Now try to relax your whole body downward and rest your head on your arms or extend them out in front of you. Give this one time to work. Try to relax feeling the stretch in your right hip. I know it's hard.

The key to this exercise is to adjust the position so that it is appropriate for your level of flexibility. You should feel the stretch in your hip and buttock and not in your knee. If this hurts your knee, adjust the position by bringing your foot down more. Also try to keep your hips square. There will be a tendency to roll toward your right. You may also place a small folded towel under your right hip for support. Try to keep your left foot flat pointing directly backward.

Relax for one minute. Repeat on the opposite side.

Pillow Squeezes on Chair

Sit upright in a hard-bottomed chair with your feet pointing straight ahead and hip-width apart. Place a small pillow or cushion between your knees. Your hands are in your lap, palms up; this helps to keep your shoulders back. With your back remaining straight, gently and evenly squeeze the pillow between your knees. Hold for a few seconds, then release. Along with strengthening the muscles inside your thighs, you may notice that every time you squeeze, your pelvis tilts forward slightly reintroducing more arch into your back. This is what we want with this exercise.

Work up to forty squeezes.

Reaching Down Under

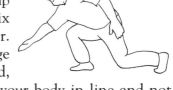

What we're doing here is mimicking the movement of reaching out one hand to pick up a fallen object under a table. Stand five or six feet away from a table with your feet together. Imagine an object has fallen just under the edge of the table. Step forward on one leg, bend, and pretend to grab the object. Try to keep your body in line and not swinging out to one side or the other. Once you have touched the spot where the imaginary object was, return to your starting position with your feet together.

Do ten of these, stepping forward with the right leg; then do ten using the other leg. Work your way up until you can do twenty on each side.

It may be difficult to do even one to begin with. The front of your thigh may quiver; your buttock muscles may feel tight; you may feel as if your knees are going to give way. Welcome to the club. Do the best you can. If this is too difficult, try lunging forward toward a higher object such as a low tabletop.

Side Crunches

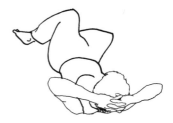

Lie on your back on the floor with your knees bent and your feet placed a comfortable distance from your bottom. Allow your knees and legs to fall toward the floor to the right side. Ideally, your right knee should touch the floor with your left knee resting on top of your right knee. If this is terribly uncomfortable, you may place a small pillow under your right knee for support.

Now place your hands on either side of your head and lift upward toward the ceiling and slightly toward the left. Hold for a second and then come down. Your head and neck should only come off the floor a few inches. Try to avoid overly tensing the muscles in your neck and shoulders. Instead, concentrate on lifting using your abdominal muscles.

Work your way up to doing twenty five of these. Varying the direction you lift slightly works different aspects of the abdominal muscles. Repeat on the opposite side.

Side-Lying Leg Lifts

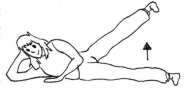

Lie on the right side of your body. Your right elbow is bent with your hand supporting your head. Make sure your body is in one plane (or as close as possible). You don't want your bottom sticking out backward, or your body to be tilted in either direction. Lift your uppermost leg straight toward the ceiling, as high as you comfortably can without altering your alignment. Your toes remain pointed in the same direction as the front of your body.

Do twenty of these or until you begin to alter your alignment. Repeat on the opposite side.

Side Sitting

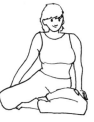

Sit on the floor with your knees bent and your legs lying on the floor to the right side. Your right foot points outward, and your left foot touches your right thigh. Try to keep your back vertical, your shoulders level, and both of your sitting bones touching the floor. It's important that you keep your back and chest as close to vertical as possible because you want the stretch in your hips and not to be absorbed by bending your body. You should feel this stretch in your right outer hip and back.

Hold for up to three minutes and then switch sides.

This exercise stretches the muscles on the outside of the hips and back, demanding your hips to open up equally on both sides. You'll probably find that one side is markedly tighter than the other. *If this exercise hurts your knees, don't do it.*

As a variation, you can add a twist to this exercise. Do the exercise close to a railing or corner of a room. Once you are in position, twist reaching behind you toward your right and grasp onto the railing with your right hand. This makes it easy to "crank" the twist and also to assure you stay vertical.

Sitting Forward Bend

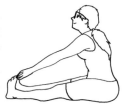

Sit on the floor with your legs extended directly in front of you. Your thighs are parallel, and your feet point toward the ceiling. Sit up straight lifting your chest and arching your back slightly. Next, extend your arms forward toward your toes. If you can grasp your toes, fine. If not, use a towel or strap to reach your toes. Focus on extending your body outward toward your toes rather than collapsing down. We don't care how far down you can go in this exercise. Only bend as far forward as you can while maintaining that small arch in your back. *Don't round your back forward to try to reach your toes.* We are trying to improve the forward bending ability of our pelvis here while providing a stretch to our hamstrings and low back. Keep your legs straight. You should feel the stretch in the backs of your legs and the front of your groins. Stretch for fifteen seconds.

Squats

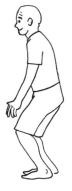

Before you say you can't do these, read the instructions carefully. Stand with your feet hip-width apart and pointing straight ahead. Bend your knees and squat down slightly so that you feel it in the fronts of your thighs. Lower yourself down a distance that is appropriate for you while challenging yourself. At first, lowering only a short distance may be enough. Don't allow your knees to flare out to either side—make sure they remain pointing straight ahead. Focus on keeping a slight arch in your back, that is, your bottom sticking out slightly as if you are about to sit down on a chair. Try to keep your torso close to vertical and not falling or rounding forward.

Hold for fifteen seconds, then come up, rest, and repeat.

As you get stronger, while focusing on the above instructions, you can go down deeper until your thighs are close to parallel with the floor.

Stair Drop

Stand with just the balls of your feet (feet pointing straight ahead) on the edge of a stair so that your heels drop downward but don't touch the lower stair. Gently hold onto the railing or wall with one or both hands just to keep your balance. Don't let your pelvis collapse forward or backward, but rather extend and lengthen upward while allowing your heels to drop down. Lift your shoulders up, then back, and down so that you position them properly. As you let your heels relax downward, you should feel a stretch in the back of your calves extending up toward your buttocks.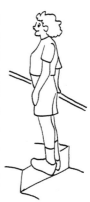

Hold for two minutes, working up to three minutes. Keep a close eye on your alignment. Watch your feet; they will want to turn in or out.

Standing Airplane

This one is a little harder and combines core strength with balance. Stand with your feet hip-width apart and pointing straight ahead. Concentrate your weight on your right foot. Now, in one smooth movement bend forward lifting your left foot off the ground and extending it directly backward. Your hands 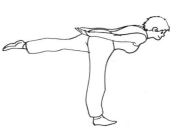 lift up to your sides with your palms pointing downward. Open up and lift your chest slightly. Focus on your alignment. Try to keep everything lifted without any sag in your low back. Keep your standing leg straight. Spreading your toes slightly on your standing foot helps with balance. You are now ready for takeoff.

Hold for fifteen to thirty seconds. Repeat using the other leg.

Standing Bent-Knee Chair Twist

This is one of my favorite exercises for regaining the twist in our hips and flanks. Set a hard-bottomed chair at about a forty-five degree angle and about three feet away from an outside corner in a room or at a doorway. Stand facing the chair and place your right foot up on the chair. Keep your hips square,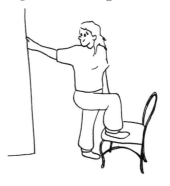

that is, keep them pointing in the direction of the back of the chair. Your left foot remains pointed straight ahead. Next, turn to your right, reach behind you, and place your hand against the wall or gently hold onto the doorway.

This is where you may have to adjust the position of the chair—both the angle and the distance—to get the right stretch for you. Your outstretched arm should be straight and at shoulder level. Without bending or tilting your hips, concentrate on opening your right shoulder outward. You may also gently push against your right outer knee with your left hand to rotate your hips in the opposite direction. Lift upward. You should feel the stretch in your right shoulder, buttock, and groin.

Hold for one minute and repeat on the other side. The key to this stretch is to adjust the position of the chair to maximize the stretch for you.

Standing Leg Balance

Stand with your feet hip-width apart. Lift your right knee and gently grasp it with your hands. Balance. Try to keep your back straight and upright and not tilted to either side. Hold for one minute. If you lose your balance and fall over, try again until the minute is up. Repeat on the other side.

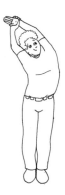

Standing Side Stretch

Stand with your feet together and pointing straight ahead. Take a moment to adjust your posture. Is your weight balanced on both feet? Do you feel centered? Lift your arms above your head grasping your left wrist with your right hand. Now, lean toward the right trying to keep your upper body in the same plane as your legs, that is, don't allow your body to fold forward or bend backward. You want to feel the stretch on the left side of your body. Find the right stretch for you and hold. Then after fifteen seconds or so, try to stretch a little farther.

Repeat on the opposite side.

Table Stretch

This exercise counteracts the tendency to hunch and roll our shoulders forward and also allows us to regain some movement in our pelvis. Find a table, desk, counter, chair, or railing; something waist height works best. Your feet are hip-width apart 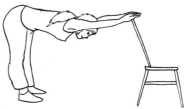 and pointing straight ahead. Lean forward and rest your hands palms down on the table. You want your legs and your torso to form a ninety-degree angle. You may have to adjust your position to get it just right. Relax. Let your head fall forward between your shoulders and let your shoulders relax. Let gravity do the work. You should feel this exercise in your shoulders, upper back, and also possibly in the hamstring area. Adjust your position so that you feel an appropriate stretch for you. By moving your bottom backward you can accentuate the stretch in your hamstrings.

Hold for one minute and eventually two minutes.

As a variation, you can try turning your hands palms upward or as close as possible. This helps open up tight muscles in the shoulders and upper back even more.

Thigh Lifts

This exercise isolates and works the muscles that flex your hips. Lie on your back with your knees bent and your feet a comfortable distance from your body. Your arms rest at your 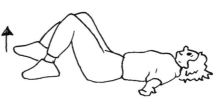 sides. Lift your right foot four inches off the ground and then lower it back down. Let the muscle deep in your groin do the work and don't use your hands to push into the ground.

Do twenty of these and then switch sides. Work up to doing forty on each side.

Toe Raises (3 parts)

1. Stand up straight alongside something you can hold on to like a counter. Your feet are together and point straight ahead; try to keep your feet, ankles, knees, and thighs touching or close to it. Lift straight up onto your toes as high as you can, then slowly lower back down. Avoid leaning to one side or the other. Work up to twenty repetitions.

2. Turn your toes inward (pigeon-toed) so that your toes are touching and your heels are about six inches apart. Lift and lower, working up to twenty repetitions.

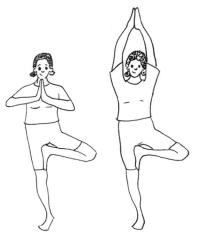

3. Turn your toes outward about six inches apart and place your heels together like a ballerina. Lift up on your toes and then lower. Work up to doing twenty of these.

Tree

This is a classic yoga posture. Stand with your feet together. Shift your weight to your left leg. Bend your right leg and place your right foot on the inside of your left thigh. If you can't get it up to your thigh, place your foot on your calf but not directly on the knee joint. Place your hands in the center of your chest in "prayer" position. Let your shoulders relax down. Try to work on rotating your right knee outward away from the center of your body, and on keeping your shoulders and hips square. You want them to be level and not rotated.

Practice this pose for one minute. If you lose your balance, try again until the whole minute is up. Repeat on the other side.

Once you are able to stand for a full minute without falling, practice raising your hands together above your head with your index fingers together and the rest of your fingers crossed. Progress until you are able to do this for one minute.

Triangle

This is a classic yoga pose. Stand with your feet about three and one half feet apart and your toes pointing straight ahead. Lift your arms to shoulder level. Your wrists should be approximately above your ankles. Turn your right foot out ninety degrees and your left foot in forty-five degrees. The heel of your right foot should line up with the arch of your left foot. Bend sideways at the waist, bringing your right hand down toward your right ankle. If you can, touch your fingers to the floor at the outside of your foot. Otherwise, grab onto your right ankle or calf. Another alternative is to place a small block to the outside of your foot and hold onto that. Keep your legs straight and only bend as far as you can while maintaining straight legs. Your left arm lifts above your head, pointing straight toward the ceiling. You can turn your head and look toward your left hand or simply look straight ahead. *Focus on opening your topmost hip up and outward* rather than collapsing or bending forward.

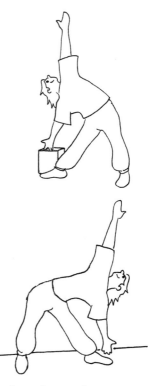

Hold for fifteen to thirty seconds, then come up slowly and repeat on the opposite side.

As a variation or if you are just starting out, do your triangle pose alongside a wall. Stand with your back to the wall. Spread your legs three and one half feet apart. Turn your left foot out ninety degrees and your right foot in forty-five degrees. Your right heel should be close to the wall and left foot a few inches away. Bend toward the left, keeping your pelvis and back against the wall as much as possible. Grab your ankle or as far down as you can while keeping both legs straight. Attempt to keep your body in the same plane as the wall, that is, bending and opening up to the side and upward rather then bending forward. Lift your right arm up so that the back of your hand touches the wall. Turn your head and look up toward your right hand if you can. Adjust your position to maximize the stretch along the sides of your body.

Hold for fifteen to thirty seconds, then come up slowly and repeat on the opposite side.

Wall Bench

Find a comfortable wall. Stand with your back toward the wall and your feet pointing straight ahead and hip-width apart. Lean back against the wall. Slide your back down the wall and keep your feet forward so that you are sitting in the air with your lower back and shoulders pressed against the wall. Your knees should be slightly behind or above your ankles forming approximately a ninety-degree angle, but not forward of your ankles. If this position is too painful on your knees, slide up the wall a little.

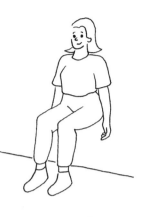

Your goal is to work your way up to holding this position for two minutes. At first fifteen seconds may be enough. The fact that this is so hard for so many of us to do means we need it.

Warrior II

Another classic yoga posture. Stand with your feet three and a half to four feet apart. Your right foot points ninety degrees to the right; your left foot is at a forty-five degree angle with the arch of your left foot in line with the heel of your right foot. Lift your arms up in line with your body. Now, extend toward the right so that your right

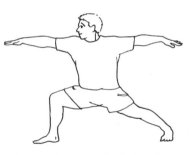

knee bends while your left leg remains straight and extended. Look out over your extended right hand. Relax your neck and shoulders. Over time try to sink down deeper until your right knee approaches a ninety-degree angle. Your knee should remain above or behind your foot and ankle, but not in front of it (not good for the knee ligaments). Stretch for fifteen seconds and then repeat on the opposite side.

Wide-Leg Forward Bend

Spread your feet so that they are three and a half to four feet apart and pointing straight ahead. Lift your arms, stretching them out to the side— your wrists should be approximately above your ankles. Now,

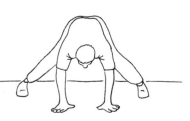

bend forward at the waist keeping your back flat and touch your hands to the floor. Protect your back when you bend forward by keeping a slight arch in your back and bracing yourself using your abdominal and core muscles. Your hips should be level—one shouldn't be higher or more forward the other. While keeping your legs straight, adjust your position so that you feel a stretch deep in your hamstrings extending up into your buttocks. If you can't reach anywhere near the floor, place a small block or stool in front of you, reach down, and hold on to that. Be careful and stay in control. Once you are down, you can move slightly from side to side to stretch tight areas. Moving your bottom backward and upward accentuates the stretch.

Stretch for thirty seconds.

Our minds affect our bodies. Our bodies affect our minds. In the next chapter, we'll look at some of these connections ...

CHAPTER 14

Bodymind

Mens sano in coporo sano
A sound mind in a sound body

—Roman

Throughout the nineties mind-body medicine came into its own. It became generally accepted that the way we think, the way we represent things to ourselves, has an effect on the health of our bodies, in some cases, even altering the progression of certain types of cancer and heart disease.

> Our minds—the ways we think and represent things to ourselves—can have a significant effect on our health.

But the converse has always remained equally true. The health of our bodies including our muscles and joints, our posture, and amount of movement we get in our lives also significantly affects our minds and emotions. There is often a tendency to underestimate the importance of this. For many of us who live busy lives, exercise seems a luxury or a waste of time. Far from it.

> Our posture and the amount of movement we get in our lives affects our minds and emotions.

Posture And Emotion

Like it or not, we both judge others and are judged by our posture and the way we move. People with more erect posture are perceived as younger, happier, more confident, and in control. How we stand, walk, and move affects how others relate to us.

How we stand and move also affects how *we* feel. It may be fair to say that when our posture is more erect, we *feel* younger, happier, more confident, and in control.

> *This is my "depressed stance." When you're depressed, it makes a lot of difference how you stand. The worst thing you can do is straighten up and hold your head high because then you'll start to feel better. If you're going to get any joy out of being depressed, you've got to stand like this.*
>
> —Charlie Brown, "Peanuts"

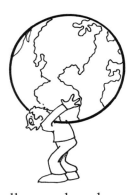

How do depressed people generally stand and move? How do they hold their shoulders and backs? What about their heads? When we're depressed or down, our bodies begin to look depressed and down. Our shoulders round forward. We round our backs as if we have the weight of the world on them. Our bodies and our worlds collapse and close in on ourselves. Our heads and eyes drop downward. We slump. We move slowly. We slouch and shuffle.

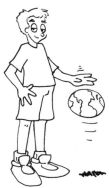

And how do we generally stand and move if we're happy or "up." That's right, we're more upright, right? We naturally tend to pull our shoulders back, lift and open our chests, and raise our heads and look more forward. We walk with more purpose.

We make assessments of people's emotions based on their posture and the way they move. Slow-moving, slouching—we know one of our co-workers is feeling out of sorts.

The curious thing is that if you make yourself assume the posture of a depressed person and walk around that way ...well, you begin to feel depressed. And if you want to feel happy and confident, throw your shoulders back, lift your chest and head, and walk that way.

If by just altering our posture for a short period of time can change how we feel, the question arises: Is it possible that poor posture may be contributing to at least some of the current epidemic of depression? Is it possible that, by correcting our posture, there is a similar restorative effect on our psyches? Lots of people think so.

Some carry this a step farther assigning emotive states to each posture disparity. Consider the answers to these questions—

- Are stiff people more set in their perceptions?
- Are flexible people more flexible and open to new ideas?
- Do people whose posture is out-of-line feel more out of sorts generally than those who are aligned?
- Are older people more set in their ways in part because they are physically stiffer? Or is a part of the aging process the accumulation of these physical and mental holdings, which make us stiff?
- Are twisted people twisted in their thinking?

Fun to think about, huh?

We Need To Move

It's written into our genetic material. We need to move. We are animals. Movement is linked to the overall health of our bodies. Motion keeps every part of our body functional. Motion also exercises our ...brains. Numerous nerve and biochemical connections link the movements of our arms and legs with our brains allowing the release of neurotransmitters, which positively affect our minds and emotions.

Sitting in one place for long periods of time or doing the same repetitive movements year after year after year contribute to the stupefaction of our minds as well as our bodies.

> Movement has an overall positive effect on our minds and emotions.

> Sad, depressed, worried? Get out and do something physical.

Our mothers and grandmothers knew this in their own way—

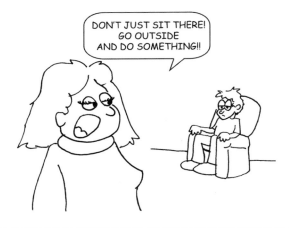

Disconnect

As we grow older, there is a tendency to become disconnected from our bodies. They are down there, and we are up here. We may know we hurt or can't do what we used to, but we often lose much of our kinesthetic sense that tells us exactly what is going on or how or where things may be beginning to go awry. Like executives stuck in the corporate office, we may not be fully aware of exactly what is going on down on the factory floor.

At our workplace our bodies are demanded to work whether they want to or not. Even if we go to the gym or work out, we may just put our bodies through their paces without ever being fully in touch with them, or only on the fringes. We run on the treadmill while reading a book, listening to music, or watching TV. We exercise while thinking of a host of other things.

Many of our role models for sports, for men in particular, also encourage a disconnect—big, bulky guys who play through pain and hardly know what they feel except that they need to pop a few more pain pills. Our sports programs encourage strength, power, aggression, and winning. The body was often a captive participant working toward these goals; it is molded, coerced, forced, and manipulated toward the goals of coaches and teams.

And because of this—

> We often haven't treated ourselves kindly, listened very well, and hence have lost touch with our bodies.

Part of the message of this book includes rekindling a gentle, conscious connection with ourselves. Yoga is great for this. Practicing any of the exercises in this book in a quiet environment helps one to become more aware of the subtle workings of your own body. Take the time when you exercise to listen to your body, to feel what *you* are feeling. Feel where you are tight, notice where you are weak. Over time, your kinesthetic sense will be restored and become more refined.

As this kinesthetic sense returns, you will become your own teacher. You will be able to tell where you are tight, stiff, weak, or out-of-line, and you will be able to know what works and how to remedy it. Another benefit of rekindling this kinesthetic sense is that you will be less likely to injure yourself by inattention.

Locked-Up Emotions

Many bodywork therapies believe that we carry or hold emotions in our bodies. At a time of trauma or significant emotion, we tighten up parts of our body and often that tightening or those constrictions persist. Over time, our bodies become the repositories of all the significant emotions we have felt throughout our lives.

> We hold emotions in our body.

As we release tight tissues, it is not uncommon to re-feel some of these emotions as they are freed and come bubbling to the surface. Re-aligning ourselves and regaining strength and flexibility becomes a form of therapy for our psyches.

My right hip has always been tighter than my left. Once while doing a deep stretch and getting nowhere, I asked myself, "Why won't my right hip let go?" And what came to me as a wave of emotion was the sensation of tightening my right buttock muscle as a small boy being spanked.

Some of the delay in regaining lost flexibility may be due to not being quite ready to let go of things emotionally. Part of stretching is a process of continually telling ourselves that we are safe, and it's okay to relax, let go, and release things.

Energy

> *I sing the body electric.*
>
> —Walt Whitman

We are all vortexes of energy. Our atoms and molecules are constantly in flux, changing, moving, flying off in all directions and being replaced by new ones. We have been called energetic patterns that perpetuate themselves. The energetic blueprint, which is ourselves, vibrates with energy.

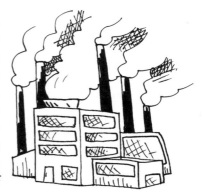

In the West our bodies are often described as machines or factories. Our hearts are pumps. Our lungs are huge bellows. Our muscles and joints comprise an intricate array of levers and pulley systems. Our energy output—our horsepower, as it were—is directly related to the efficiency of the running of each of these component parts. And just as when a machine breaks down, when we break down, we think of having to fix the machine.

Eastern medicine and yoga provide a somewhat different description. It describes us as energy fields. When we are sick, our energy is blocked of not flowing properly. Acupuncture, acupressure, yoga, and Oriental medicine speak of *energy blockages*. In effect, we want to remove our blockages, freeing up the energy that is already ours.

In the Eastern viewpoint, we aren't creating new energy. We are simply freeing up energy, which is already ours or already available to us. In the Western viewpoint we are making more efficient and economical use of our resources, and thus we have more energy available to do the other things we want or need to do.

Both are valid descriptions. But one thing we can be sure of—energy—that's what we're all after. We all want more of it, or at least enough of it to do what we need to get done.

Conserving The Energy We Have

> *A body whose components are symmetrically*
> *distributed around a vertical line dissipates*
> *less of its energy in meaningless movement and*
> *meaningless tensions ...In such bodies the*
> *reservoirs of available energy must stand at a*
> *higher level.*
>
> —Ida Rolf

Over millions of years at each evolutionary step of the way, our bodies have optimized our structure to limit energy expenditure. The biological mandate of our bodies has always been, "Don't do any more than you have to."

Correct posture and alignment is the anatomical equivalent of this. Ida Rolf in her book, *Rolfing*, makes the point that with improvements in our body's alignment, we intuitively sense a more economical use of resources. When we say such things as "That feels better," or "I feel great," we are sensing increased efficiency in our bodies. When our muscles are balanced in strength and flexibility, we feel a surge of well-being.

Let's say, based on the food we eat, we are each given one hundred packets of energy every day.

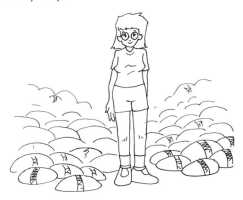

But let's say our alignment is off (we fight a continual war against gravity to stay upright), we don't use the muscles we are supposed to to do things (they are weak), and it's just generally more of a struggle or effort to get around. Maybe twenty of our energy packets are used up due to inefficiency.

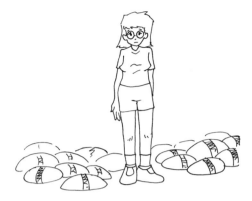

This leaves us with fewer packets of energy to do all the things we want to do. As we return our bodies toward correct alignment, as we move with more efficiency and grace, energy is freed up. And that is why we feel a surge of energy as we regain our functional movement potential.

> Any time we move our bodies toward improved
> alignment and more economy of movement, it leads
> to increased energy.

As a consequence of this, we are able to move more and we want to move more. We put ourselves on an upward spiral of activity, function, and energy.

Our Center

> *If you want to cure the soul,*
> *cure the body.*
>
> —Aristotle

Our body's center of gravity is located in the sacral region just above the tailbone. Many spiritual beliefs put the base of our soul in the same area. In fact, the word "sacrum" means sacred bone.

Our body's central region, which includes our core muscles, has significance both in our posture and our energy. Martial artists talk about our energy, *chi* or *ki*, coming from our center in the area around our umbilicus and speak of all movement being initiated from this region. In yoga philosophy, three of the seven chakras (psychic centers) are centered in the pelvic and lower abdominal region.

It has been said with regard to spiritual pursuits—first, become a good animal. A healthy body is less of an intrusion in our lives, allowing us to pursue our spiritual or worldly goals with more vigor. Don't underestimate the refinement of one's energy and intention that comes from a pain-free, functional body.

Change The Way You Think: Our minds affect our bodies; our bodies affect our minds. Posture affects our emotions. Muscle and joint health free up our energy.

Everything written so far means nothing—unless we do something. The next chapter will tell help us do that ...

CHAPTER 15

Putting It All Together

Thus, though we cannot make our sun
Stand still, yet we will make him run.

—Andrew Marvell

The message of this book is that there are things we can do—*and only we can do*—that can allow us to look younger and stay active longer. There are things that only we can do to help preserve and protect our muscles and joints.

Our health *is* one of the most important things. Not money, fame, success, or possessions. Even family and friends can pall in importance when we are incapacitated or in constant pain. Make an effort now while you can to preserve and protect your muscles and joints.

The exercises in this book are not all-inclusive. More important are the principles; your goal as you grow older has to be to stay strong, flexible, aligned, and active. There are many other similar exercises in other books. Most of them are good. Correcting one's posture, however, in particular requires a specific series of exercises similar to the ones in this book.

Some of you reading this book are on the cusp. You haven't yet experienced any precipitous decline in your muscle and joint health. For you in particular, a small effort now can make a big difference in the years to come. Doing a few exercises a day or several times a week can prevent the beginning of that slide down the downward spiral.

Once things start to deteriorate, once you get the first one or two chinks in your musculoskeletal armor, it takes considerably more effort to turn things around. And the unfortunate fact is, at that time, fewer people have the wherewithal it takes to turn things around. Many people won't make the effort now, and won't have the energy to make it later. Thus, they doom themselves to the downward spiral before their time. Do something now while you can.

> The longer you wait, the more effort it takes to turn
> things around.

The wise sage tells us that all journeys begin with that first step. Wherever you are right now, that is your starting point. It doesn't matter whether you are fat, slim, weak, strong, twisted, crooked, or broken down. It doesn't matter whether you hurt or have had previous orthopedic surgery. There are *always* things you can do to bolster up your strength, flexibility, and alignment in ways that are appropriate for you. No matter what your level of muscle and joint fitness or un-fitness, you can be assured that it will get worse if you do nothing.

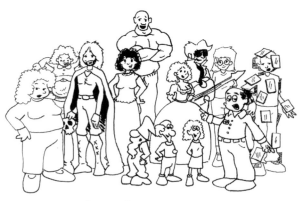

DO SOMETHING

> Develop an exercise program that includes exercises
> similar to the ones in this book that work for you.
> Do it on a regular basis.

Small Change Can Make A Difference—But More Is Better

Throughout this book, I make it a point to say that every little bit helps.

One or two exercises may be enough to strengthen a weak muscle and take pressure off an inflamed joint. Improving your posture only slightly may be enough to markedly improve your appearance and allow you to keep doing activities you would have otherwise given up. Small changes in your beliefs may allow you to keep active for years to come.

> Small changes *can* make a difference.

But while true—and we like that message—the fact remains that if you are way out-of-line, stiff, and weak, it's going to take a determined effort on your part to alter the trajectory. And it's going to take time. We don't become strong, we don't regain lost flexibility, we don't alter our posture that has been that way for decades in a few weeks time.

> If you're stiff, weak, and out of alignment, it's going to take a determined, consistent effort on your part to turn things around. And it's going to take time.

And while small changes can make a difference, big changes can make a big difference. For those of you who are up to it, I encourage you to get really strong, really flexible, and correct your alignment and stay that way.

> Big changes can make a big difference.

The Future

Not your future or my future—the future of others. You and I have the ability to change the mindset of others. Children, adolescents, and young adults in this country are particularly prone to the decreasing demand for physical activity. Where children used to play outside all year, now streets, ball fields, and parks are virtually empty except for organized activities.

Muscle and joint injuries that used to be present only in older, more sedentary individuals are now showing up in children and teens. Increased weight is a continual problem both caused by and contributing to decreased activity. In schools, gym classes have become an elective. It is as if some of us may not need our bodies for the rest of our lives.

Just as such things as global warming are not without their eventual consequences, it is the same with physical activity. Lack of physical activity will eventually take its toll.

The amount and variety of physical activity that children and young adults receive form the basis on which the rest of the muscle and joint life will be played out. Peak bone formation occurs during adolescence and pre-adolescence. Lack of activity during this period can set the stage for osteoporosis later in life. Development of key muscle groups forms a repository of strength that can be drawn on later in life.

Any problems in our children's muscles and joints, any postural mal-alignments that develop during these early years will have to play themselves out over decades. If Jason has a slumped posture now, what will he be like in his twenties or thirties or even later? If Kimberly is overweight now and her knees hurt, what will her knees be like twenty years from now?

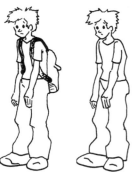

Related to this, there is a backward-type of logic that often puts the cart before the horse. For example, the problem is not that children's backpacks are necessarily too heavy. The problem is the lack of muscle development that allows them to be carried properly. Having a hunched-over, collapsed posture to begin with means that the muscles to carry a backpack in an upright position are unable to do their job. And carrying a backpack or doing anything in a hunched-over position will cause the persistence of the muscular pattern that keeps one hunched over.

For children, any and all physical activity is good. Too often Johnny only plays soccer. Matilda only plays tennis. Playing only one sport or doing only one activity often leads to imbalance of muscle strength at an early age.

The obsession with winning or being "number one" also contributes to a generation of young adults who feel "why bother."

> Sports for children are not about becoming a superstar. They are about getting in touch with your body, learning and feeling how it functions, learning its thresholds, and developing the strength, flexibility, timing, coordination, and muscle-sense you need for the rest of your lives.

> Fostering a love of physical activity is one of the
> greatest gifts you can give a child or young adult.

If you are a teacher, parent, or have any contact with children, by your example and beliefs make it a point to instill in children the importance of physical activity. Present or discuss the principles in this book.

Encouraging physical activity in all our children, regardless of their performance level, will pay great dividends in the years to come. A child who is comfortable with their body and who learns to enjoy physical activity without judgment will tend to keep being active long after the so-called "athletes" have hung up their letter jackets.

> Encourage and support physical activity in children
> and adolescents.

Final Thoughts

There are things you can do that can make a difference.

The principles and the exercises in this book can make you look younger and stay active longer.

Get and stay strong and flexible. Maintain your posture and stay active.

Most people won't do anything until things get bad enough. Then it often takes so much effort to turn things around that most people simply accept things as they are.

You will see the most dramatic gains in day-to-day activity by strengthening your core and lower extremities.

If you are doing anything to maintain your muscles and joints, you are miles ahead of most people. If you focus on correcting and maintaining your alignment as well, you are light years ahead.

Take advantage of varied activity and doing things yourself. Take advantage of classes in your community.

Control your weight.

O

Oatis, Carol, 90
Orthopedic braces, 81
Osteoporosis, 32

P

Pain, 2-3
    location of, 22
Peak bone mass, 32
Peanuts (quote), 192
Pelvis, 61-72
    backward-tilted, 51, 62-63
    forward-tilted, 51, 62
    importance in correcting
        posture, 50-52
    need for movement, 65
    side-to-side tilt, 64
Perry (quote), 73
Pilates, 96
Pilates, Joseph (quote), 149
Pirie, Gordon (quote), 103
Poor Richard's Almanack
    (quote), 35
Posture, 45-60
    effect on appearance, 45,
        54, 55
    effect on emotion, 91-93
    effects of bad posture, 54-55
    how to change, 57-58,
        119-120
    importance of, 45
    overview of correct alignment,
        47-52
    tips on changing, 122, 124
    what creates differences in, 56
*Posture Alignment, The Missing
    Link in Health and Fitness*, 60
Posture Makes Perfect, 119

Q

Quadriceps, 82
Quirks in posture, 57

R

Resistance training, 91-92
Rocky, (quote), 87
Rolf, Ida (quotes), 17, 25, 29,
    77, 197
Rolfing, 29
Roman (quote), 191

S

Science of Flexibility, 117
Shoulders, rounded, 53
Silva, Mira and Shyam Mehta,
    117
Small change, 139, 202
Spine, 150-151
    loss of height with aging, 32
    S-curve, 50, 151
Sports, 132-133
Stairs, 134
Strength, 87-96
    downward spiral, 89
    importance of, 87-96
Stretching, 109
    keys to effective stretching,
        110-112
*Strong Men and Women Beat
    Arthritis*, 147
Symmetry, 20

T
Tendons, 34
Tensegrity, 20
Therapeutic Exercise, 45

U-V
Victim mentality, 131

W-X
Walden, Patricia, 117
Wear and Tear, 147
Weight, 35-36, 85
Weight lifting, 94-95
Whitman, Walt (quote), 196
Wright, Stephen (quote), 74

Y-Z
Yoga, 115-116
Yoga for Beginners, 117
Yoga, The Iyengar Way, 117

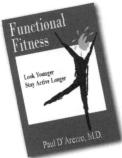

ORDER FUNCTIONAL FITNESS NOW

Please send me _____copies of *Functional Fitness— Look Younger, Stay Active Longer* at $19.95 plus $1.00 shipping and handling media mail (4-14 days delivery) or $3.95 priority mail (2-3 days delivery). Add $.50 shipping for each additional book. Colorado residents add 2.9 % sales tax.

ORDER POSTURE ALIGNMENT NOW

Please send me _____copies of *Posture Alignment— The Missing Link in Health and Fitness* at $19.95 plus $1.00 shipping and handling media mail (4-14 days delivery) or $3.95 priority mail (2-3 days delivery). Add $.50 shipping for each additional book. Colorado residents add 2.9 % sales tax.

My check or money order for _____ is enclosed.

Name   _____
Address   _____
City/State/Zip _____
Phone   _____

Please make check payable and return this form to:

Marcellina Mountain Press
PO Box 6781
Colorado Springs, CO 80934

For credit card orders call: 1-800-431-1579
Or visit our website: www.posturealignment.com
Retailers or distributors, please contact us for discounts.